A MAJOR DRUG COMPANY MADE $1.2 BILLION FROM PROZAC IN ONE YEAR. BUT WHAT IS ITS COST TO YOU?!

* The maker, Eli Lilly, insists Prozac is safe, but there is an avalanche of lawsuits against the company and physicians who have prescribed it.

* Fans of the drug say it can make "normal" people feel better than they ever have . . . BUT there are hundreds of cases of users who became emotionally disturbed, or committed suicide or murder while on Prozac.

* Prozac is taken for "winter blues," obesity, anorexia, bulimia, phobia, anxiety, panic disorder, chronic fatigue syndrome, PMS, post-partum depression, drug and alcohol addiction, migraines, arthritis, and behavioral problems in children . . . BUT the FDA approved it only for depression and obsessive-compulsive disorder.

* The drug company says there are no long-term effects from Prozac . . . BUT clinical trials lasted only six weeks.

* Prozac has been praised for making its users "less sensitive" . . . BUT it also makes them less in-touch with reality, less caring, and less loving.

"An urgently needed book."
—*Anderson Valley Advertiser*

"Breggin has long stood for speaking the truth . . . He is a one-man intellectual SWAT team."
—*Jeffrey Moussaieff Mason, Ph.D.*
author of *The Assault on Truth* and *Final Analysis*

TALKING BACK TO PROZAC

WHAT DOCTORS WON'T TELL YOU ABOUT TODAY'S MOST CONTROVERSIAL DRUG

PETER R. BREGGIN, M.D.
AND
GINGER ROSS BREGGIN

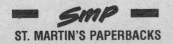
ST. MARTIN'S PAPERBACKS

Illustration on page 25 copyright © 1994 by Durell Godfrey.

TALKING BACK TO PROZAC

Copyright © 1994 by Peter R. Breggin, M.D., and Ginger Ross Breggin.

Author photo by Ginger Ross Breggin.

Library of Congress Catalog Card Number: 94-12572

ISBN: 0-312-95606-1

Printed in the United States of America

St. Martin's Press hardcover edition/June 1994
St. Martin's Paperbacks edition/September 1995

10 9 8 7 6 5 4 3 2 1

To Phil and Jean Ross,
Our Loving Parents

Contents

NINE
How and Why to Stop Taking Psychiatric Drugs
213

TEN
Understanding and Overcoming Depression
228

Acknowledgments

Our assistant, Melissa Magruder, has been indispensable in copyediting and maintaining and retrieving the complex materials required for the completion of this book and in handling innumerable daily activities around the office. She has made this project run smoothly. Chad Alden joined us as an intern at precisely the moment we needed research assistance and we appreciate his generous help.

We are grateful to our friends who read portions of the manuscript, especially Kevin McCready and David Cohen, who reviewed it cover to cover, and offered many valuable suggestions. Helpful comments were made by Robert Grimm on neurological aspects and David Whitford on statistical issues. We also thank Paul Sleven for his untiring, admirable legal vetting. We, of course, remain wholly and exclusively responsible for the final product.

We wish to thank the more than one hundred members of the Board of Directors and the Advisory Council of the Center for the Study of Psychiatry. Founded more than twenty years ago by Peter Breggin, this network of medical and mental health professionals, attorneys, patient advocates, and members of Congress continues to provide enormous moral and professional support. More than two dozen board and advisory council members are psychiatrists, and another dozen are drawn from other medical specialties, including internal medicine, neurology, and pediatrics. We especially wish to acknowledge John George and Michael Valentine, co-directors of the Center's new membership division, *Children First!*

We are grateful for the mutual support we have shared with groups and individuals who identify themselves as survivors of psychiatry and psychiatric drugs. In areas related to this book, we have worked particularly closely with Guy McConnell, national director of the Prozac Survivors Support Group, Inc., and state directors Bonnie Leitsch (Kentucky), Ann Tracy (Utah), and Dwight Harlor III (Ohio).

This is the third book of ours published by St. Martin's Press, the first two being *Toxic Psychiatry* (1991) and *Beyond Conflict* (1992) by Peter Breggin. It will be followed by a fourth, *The War Against Children* (fall 1994), coauthored by Peter and Ginger Breggin. Barbara Anderson is the very competent, congenial editor of this book and we look forward to a long relationship with her.

Our agent, Richard Curtis, supported us from the beginning when it was as yet difficult to get published. Richard, thanks for your continued help!

This book is co-created, but Peter Breggin did the actual writing, and he alone is responsible for any observations or opinions on medicine, psychiatry, the FDA, psychiatric drugs, and pharmaceutical company practices. Ginger Breggin provided important concepts and directions, edited the entire manuscript several times, and organized and supervised the vast amount of activity required to develop the research and background material, to maintain the files, and to work with resource persons.

The awkward problem of how to refer to the authors in the text has been resolved by using "I" to refer to Peter Breggin, since it is to his activities as a physician and psychiatrist that the text most frequently refers. The word "we" will be used to designate both authors. Ginger Breggin will be referred to by name when describing her specific activities.

Acronyms of Organizations

AAAS—American Association for the Advancement of Science

ADAMHA—Alcohol, Drug Abuse, and Mental Health Administration (*now absorbed into NIH*)

AMA—American Medical Association

APA—American Psychiatric Association *or* American Psychological Association

CH.A.D.D.—Children with Attention-Deficit Disorders

DHHS—Department of Health and Human Services (*includes the FDA, the NIH, and the CDC*)

FAES—Foundation for Advanced Education in the Sciences

FDA—Food and Drug Administration

GAO—U.S. General Accounting Office

HHS—*same as* DHHS

NAMI—National Alliance for the Mentally Ill

NAS—National Academy of Sciences (*also see NRC*)

NIH—National Institutes of Health

NIAA—National Institute of Alcoholism and Alcohol Abuse (*formerly part of ADAMHA; now part of the NIH*)

NIDA—National Institute of Drug Abuse (*formerly part of ADAMHA; now part of the NIH*)

NIMH—National Institute of Mental Health (*formerly part of ADAMHA; now part of the NIH*)
NRC—National Research Council (*part of NAS*)
NSF—National Science Foundation
PHS—U.S. Public Health Service

How to Use This Book

First, an important warning:

> When trying to withdraw from many psychiatric drugs, patients can develop serious and even life-threatening emotional and physical reactions. In short, it is dangerous not only to *start* taking psychiatric drugs but also can be hazardous to *stop* taking them. Therefore, withdrawal from psychiatric drugs should be done under medical and clinical supervision.

Most books about psychiatric drugs provide the kind of information that drug advocates and pharmaceutical companies want the public to have. At best, they offer a watered-down version of information that is at the fingertips of most physicians and other professionals.

This book is different. It provides information not readily available, even to most experts in the field. Much of it, in fact, has been systematically withheld from physicians and patients alike. Nonetheless, this book cannot be used as a treatment handbook. We suggest instead that you share it with your personal physician or mental health professional. Almost certainly, he or she will be unfamiliar with some if not much of what it contains.

We have provided an extensive bibliography that lists every author, article, or project mentioned in the book. If the reference cannot be located easily by the name of the author, the numbered chapter note will help you find the source in the bibliography. The appendix to the book contains information on psychiatric reform organizations, self-help support groups, therapy resources, legal resources, and standard sources of drug information.

In most cases we have provided identifying information about the professionals whose work we cite in the book. Psychiatrists are physicians; they have medical degrees. As medical doctors, they have the right to prescribe medications. Some psychiatrists are also trained in psychotherapy or "talking therapy," but many of them lack these skills. While psychiatrists take leadership roles in promoting psychiatric drugs, many family physicians and other medical specialists also prescribe these medications. Psychologists are trained in a variety of disciplines, including research, psychological testing, and psychotherapy. They have Ph.D., rather than M.D., degrees and cannot prescribe medications.

Many biologically oriented psychiatrists argue that medication is the best or only approach to the problems they diagnose and treat, but there is a great diversity of opinion about this in the field of mental health and within the public. While some psychologists are lobbying for the right to prescribe medication, they have not as yet obtained this dubious power. Like many mental health professionals, however, some psychologists support the pharmacological approach that we criticize, while many others do not. In seeking help from mental health professionals—including psychiatrists, psychologists, clinical social workers, counselors, and family therapists—it is best to inquire in advance about their views on psychiatric drugs.

TALKING
BACK
TO
PROZAC

ONE

Should We Listen to Prozac?

Nearly everyone knows someone who is taking Prozac. In urban centers, where Prozac has achieved fadlike status, most people can name several friends or co-workers who are taking the medication. Among teenagers in our suburban hometown, Prozac is also a familiar drug. The youngsters tend to know many friends who are on it.

One of my patients recently told me, "Nearly everyone in my office is on it." She was experiencing peer pressure to take a prescription medication. Convinced of its safety, some people casually share their pills with friends who seem depressed.

As a recent *New York Times* headline announced, "With Millions Taking Prozac, A Legal Drug Culture Arises."[1] Columnists are joking about putting it in the drinking water.[2]

Prozac is becoming America's drug.

A BRIEF HISTORY OF PROZAC . . . OR, THE MAKING OF A MIRACLE DRUG

Currently the most widely prescribed and controversial psychiatric drug, Prozac began its life in the research laboratories of Eli Lilly & Company. A Lilly researcher named D. T. Wong published the first article about the drug in 1974. In 1975 it was given the official chemical name fluoxetine and later the company selected the trade name Prozac.

In February 1977, Dista Products Company, a division of Eli Lilly & Company, submitted a new drug application to the Food and Drug Administration (FDA) for Prozac. This initiated the lengthy approval process through the government agency. By April 1981 the FDA gave permission for Phase III, the controlled clinical trials, to begin. The trials were organized, supervised, funded, and evaluated by Lilly (chapter 3 provides a more complete discussion of these trials). They lasted through the end of 1982. In the ensuing several years, Eli Lilly and the FDA evaluated the studies and collected other information relevant to drug approval.

In October 1985, the FDA gave initial approval to Prozac. Their final approval letter was sent to Lilly in late December 1987, and Lilly began marketing the drug in January 1988. From discovery to marketing, Prozac's gestation lasted more than a dozen years. The FDA approval process lasted more than a decade. But within only a few months of its introduction for consumer use, Prozac was well on its way to fame (and fortune).

By 1989, annual sales for the drug had reached $350 million—more than the total amount previously spent annually by Americans on all antidepressants combined. At that point, Prozac already represented more than one-tenth of Lilly's $4.18 billion in annual sales.[3] Despite growing controversy about Prozac-related murder and suicide, sales of the drug in 1990 doubled over those of the previous year. At that time Lilly reported that 650,000 prescriptions were being written each month.[4]

On March 26, 1990, *Newsweek* put a huge Prozac capsule* on its cover with a subhead announcing, "A Breakthrough Drug for Depression." The story, by reporter

---

*Lilly calls the capsules by the trade name "Pulvules," which apparently designates the fact that they are slightly tapered at one end.

Geoffrey Cowley, displayed the photo of a smiling woman, captioned, "I'm nowhere near perfect, but it's a big, big improvement." Seemingly without embarrassment, *Newsweek* reported how another woman exclaimed, "I call myself Ms. Prozac." The magazine anticipated that "these breakthrough drugs may change the lives of millions." It's no coincidence that in 1991 and 1992, Prozac gave Lilly a nearly $1 billion share of the $8 billion antidepressant market.

In 1993, Prozac gained an even higher profile with the publication of psychiatrist Peter Kramer's *Listening to Prozac.* Kramer described some Prozac users as feeling "better than ever" or "more like my true self."[5] *Listening to Prozac* spent twenty-one weeks on the *New York Times* bestseller list.

Prozac's 1993 annual sales reached nearly $1.2 billion.[6] This figure represents an increasing proportion of the company's total revenues, which rose to $6 billion in that year. Toward the end of 1993, it was estimated that 6 million Americans and an additional 4 million people worldwide had taken the antidepressant, with no end in sight to the mounting numbers.

Prozac is now the most frequently prescribed psychiatric drug. Physicians, mostly non-psychiatrists, are now writing almost one million prescriptions a month for the drug, which retails in most areas for approximately $63 for a one-month, one-a-day, supply of 20 mg. capsules.[7] The recent FDA approval of Prozac for the treatment of obsessive-compulsive disorder and for bulimia will probably lead to another escalation in sales.

Prozac's newly arrived competitors have begun to vie for a share of the market in this new class of drugs called SSRIs (selective serotonin reuptake inhibitors). Zoloft, whose chemical name is sertraline, is a product of Roerig, a division of Pfizer, Incorporated. Approved by the FDA in December 1991, it reached annual sales of $195 million in 1992. Industry analysts predict it will achieve the $800 million mark by 1997. Paxil, or paroxetine, manufactured and distributed by SmithKline Beecham, was the next SSRI to receive FDA approval. Pfizer and SmithKline Beecham are both even larger than Lilly, each with annual revenues exceeding $7 billion. These three giants are Fortune 500 companies and have the capacity to exert considerable influence upon the medical and psychiatric professions; state and federal governments, including both houses of Congress; print and electronic media; the public; and, as we shall see, even the court system.

Two other Prozac-like SSRIs are coming into the marketplace. Luvox (fluvoxamine) has recently been approved by the FDA for obsessive-compulsive disorder and is already in use in Canada and elsewhere as an antidepressant. Serzone (nefazadone) is undergoing FDA approval for depression.

Once a drug is approved for marketing by the FDA, there are no government controls over what the physician can prescribe it for. While Prozac was originally approved for depression—and only recently for obsessive-compulsive disorder—it and the other SSRIs quickly began to be prescribed for a wide variety of ailments and difficulties, such as seasonal affective disorder (SAD) or "winter blues," obesity, anorexia, bulimia, phobia, anxiety and panic disorder, chronic fatigue syndrome, premenstrual syndrome (PMS), post-partum depression, drug and alcohol addiction, migraine headaches, arthritis, body dysmorphic disorder (BBD),[8] and, finally, behavioral and emotional problems in children and adolescents.

With the publication of Peter Kramer's book, Prozac entered a new phase. It became a drug for enhancing the lives of people who otherwise consider themselves normal. Super qualities that users and addicts typically attribute to illicit or recreational drugs, from alcohol to cocaine, began to be attributed to Prozac.

The winter of 1993–1994 saw a new explosion of promotion and controversy surrounding Prozac as well as Zoloft and Paxil. Riding on the success of *Listening to Prozac*, on February 7, 1994, *Newsweek* published yet another major story on the pill by Geoffrey Cowley. Emblazoned on the cover was "Beyond Prozac," and the cover copy captured the nation's new preoccupation—Prozac for personality enhancement:

SHY?
FORGETFUL?
ANXIOUS?
FEARFUL?
OBSESSED?

HOW SCIENCE
WILL LET YOU
CHANGE YOUR
PERSONALITY
WITH A PILL

A series of extraordinarily laudatory TV news stories followed. One of them, billed as an exposé, trooped a series of grinning Prozac consumers across the screen. As the only criticism, the show's analyst wondered if there wasn't something inherently immoral about a drug that was so wonderful. Another show raised the question of unfairness. Because of their increased alertness and drive, weren't Prozac users getting an unfair advantage in the business world? Would everyone feel compelled to take it just to keep up with the competition?

At first, serious criticism and critics were absent from the pro-drug media hype for Prozac. But the daytime talk shows soon began to discover the existence of the darker undercurrent that had been missed by the TV news camera, including large numbers of people who said that they or their family members had been emotionally damaged and even ruined or killed by the drug.

By this time I had gained visibility as an outspoken critic of Prozac and other psychiatric drugs, and I found myself being invited onto so many talk shows, including *Oprah,* that I couldn't schedule appearances on all of them. Meanwhile, the usual flurries of print media inquiries had turned into an avalanche at our nonprofit research and educational institute, the Center for the Study of Psychiatry.

The Prozac controversy reached ludicrous heights in early 1994 when psychologist James D. Goodwin gained national recognition as the "Pied Piper of Prozac," amid charges brought against him by his state psychology board that claimed he was diagnosing patients too quickly and was too often recommending Prozac. Since starting his practice of clinical psychology in the Apple Capital of the World, the small town of Wenatchee, Washington, Goodwin has referred 700 to 800 patients to physicians for the prescription of Prozac.[9]

When Peter Kramer and I appeared on Oprah Winfrey's television talk show on March 7, 1994, Goodwin was seen from Wenatchee via satellite with a roomful of adoring Prozac patients. Goodwin presented a twelve-year-old girl who seemed to recite prepared statements as to how the drug had saved her. Other of his patients came to Chicago to be on the show and joined a large group of Prozac users, many of whom seemed both euphoric and hostile. It struck me, and I suggested on *Oprah*, that Goodwin was leading what's tantamount to a Prozac cult.

In a March 3, 1994, Associated Press release, writer Aviva Brandt began her story by noting that Goodwin had been "accused of urging the antidepressant drug too forcefully on patients and without adequate evaluation of their condition." She then continued, in obvious dismay, "It took him 15 minutes to suggest I try Prozac to relieve what he called a 'mild form of depression.' "

Goodwin states that he himself has been taking Prozac for years. Some people taking Prozac, as we shall document, develop social insensitivity, lack of judgment, and self-destructive, grandiose claims and actions.

Recently Eli Lilly began to show concern about the growing tendency to advocate Prozac as a personality enhancer.[10] In a full-page ad in the March 18, 1994, *Psychiatric News*, the official newspaper of the American

Psychiatric Association, the drug company decried "trivializing a serious illness" in the media. The ad asserted, "Much of this attention has trivialized the very serious nature of the disease Prozac was specifically developed to treat—*clinical depression.*"

Psychiatrists justify using antidepressants on the grounds that depression is a biochemical disorder. Perhaps Lilly feared that the medical aura surrounding the drug was being discredited by overly enthusiastic advocates. The company may also have feared that people would begin to take seriously the comparison I was making in the media between Prozac and classical stimulants, such as amphetamines and cocaine.

Is Wenatchee, Washington, merely an exaggerated microcosm of America's enthusiastic acceptance of Prozac? Is *Brave New World* a real possibility? What is the tradeoff, mentally and morally, when a person seems to feel better on any drug and on Prozac in particular? What does Prozac do to the capacity for empathy and love? To self-reflection? What does it mean to be "euphoric," and are there gradations of euphoria too subtle for most doctors and patients to recognize? How does drug euphoria differ from genuine happiness?

The Prozac craze at first suggests a radical change in America's thinking and even in public policy. It used to be that we suspected and even vilified drugs that "just made you feel good." The government outlawed them. And does this enthusiasm for Prozac suggest problems with the drug that we haven't yet faced?

Gradually, the media and the public are becoming aware of potentially dangerous implications in the popularity of this new drug. As a result of the avalanche of adverse publicity, including medical and media reports of violence and suicide, the FDA felt compelled to hold hearings on Prozac in 1991.

Dozens of Prozac survivors, their families, and friends, traveled from across the country to give five-minute accounts of their painful and sometimes deadly encounters with the drug. Nancy Veasey, a registered nurse in Philadelphia, testified to the FDA committee:

> In September of 1990 an article appeared in the *Philadelphia Enquirer*. As a result of that, the Prozac Survivors Group in the Philadelphia area was launched.... I met and talked with by phone 15 people directly and indirectly affected by the drug, not a very impressive group, but what is impressive is that out of the 15 there are five deaths recorded in my notes. These are the facts.
>
> A 36-year-old mother of two, while on Prozac, attempted suicide by impulsively ingesting a toxic dose of medication.
>
> A 42-year-old man watched helplessly as his 36-year-old wife casually, with no warning, picked up a knife and cut both her wrists while on Prozac.
>
> A 50-year-old man with some memory impairment struggles today to express the devastating and long-lasting effect of this drug.
>
> A 49-year-old man, while on Prozac, blacked out while driving and was involved in a car accident.
>
> A 71-year-old man shot himself seven days after being prescribed Prozac, one week before his daughter's wedding.
>
> A 58-year-old man, while on Prozac, developed violent behavior directed toward his sister, his primary caretaker. He was hospitalized. He has since died.
>
> The mother of a 40-year-old Harvard physician found her daughter dead. On the nightstand was a bottle labeled Prozac. The coroner's report showed excessive amounts of Prozac in the blood. Just three months ago, upon receiving her daughter's effects, her grief-stricken husband died. Needless to say, this is one woman who is literally immobilized by grief, as I am sure many others here today are.
>
> In June of this year a woman found her husband dead by hanging in the basement of their home one week after Prozac was prescribed for him. There were no signs or warning signals. He simply got up, as he did frequently at

night, and went downstairs and hung himself. His son cannot go down there to this day.

In an interview with Ginger Breggin, Nancy explained that Prozac had adversely affected a family member, leading her to seek contact with other survivors of Prozac, and ultimately to become a leader in the reform movement.

Prozac's horizon is full of storm warnings—including many tragedies that have already struck. In addition to the more dramatic cases of murder and suicide attributed to Prozac that have made the news, Eli Lilly declared in its 1992 annual report to the Securities and Exchange Commission that in "approximately 170 actions, plaintiffs seek to recover damages as a result of the ingestion of Prozac." It adds, "in the opinion of the company, such actions will not ultimately result in any liability that would have a material adverse effect on its consolidated financial position."[11]

A 1990 report by Natalie Angier in the *New York Times* confirms that most of the suits against Lilly are related to violent behavior and thoughts, suicidal obsessions and acts, and self-mutilation. That most of the suits against Lilly involve allegations of violent or self-destructive behavior is further confirmed by my discussions and consultations with attorneys and clients who have brought suits or are initiating new ones against the drug company.

The suits against Lilly entail product liability in which the company is charged with failing to test the drug properly and failing to give proper warning of its adverse side effects,* as well as negligence in regard to making, marketing, or promoting Prozac. The allegations often hinge on the drug company's promotional materials, specifically whether or not they sufficiently warn doctors, patients,

---

*Not all drug side effects are necessarily negative or dangerous, but for ease of communication, adverse effects and side effects will be used synonymously.

and the public about drug-induced mental aberrations, including violence against self and others. As of now, to our knowledge none of these suits have come to trial.

The suits against Eli Lilly are only a portion of the legal actions being generated by Prozac. Dozens of malpractice suits—the total number is unknown, but attorneys estimate that it is very large—have been brought against physicians for alleged negligence in prescribing Prozac. According to lawyers involved in some of these cases, most of them also concern drug-induced violence and suicide. Many of these legal actions involve both malpractice and product liability resulting from the same patient's treatment.

In yet another court activity involving Prozac, people who were taking Prozac when they committed crimes are defending themselves in the criminal justice system on the grounds that Prozac caused or contributed to their actions. We shall learn more about these various kinds of suits throughout the book.

Meanwhile, I know firsthand that the number of those suits is growing and that the major ones have yet to be decided by a jury. No other psychiatric medication has ever generated such an outpouring of legal responses within its first few years on the market. There is nothing comparable. Not since amphetamines were used as antidepressants years ago has any antidepressant been so consistently and repeatedly associated with violence and suicide.

It is striking that, with all the publicity about Prozac, few professionals or patients have come forward to describe similar effects from other antidepressants.* There has been no bandwagon effect. In my speeches, consultations, and workshops, for example, new stories about

---

*Perhaps because of more limited experience with Paxil or Zoloft or perhaps because of subtle pharmacological differences from Prozac, there have been far fewer reports of adverse behavioral reactions in association with Zoloft and Paxil.

Prozac and violence or suicide frequently come up, but similar reports rarely turn up in association with other classes of antidepressants.

AN UNDERGROUND MOVEMENT OF VICTIMS

While many patients and professionals seem to be listening to Prozac—that is, to its manufacturer, Eli Lilly, and to the medical-industrial complex that promotes medication—a hitherto underground movement of Prozac survivors is making an increasing public impact. Guy McConnell of Clovis, California, is president of the Prozac Survivors Support Group, a national organization previously directed by Louisville, Kentucky, resident Bonnie Leitsch, who became suicidal while taking Prozac.

The members of the national Prozac Survivors Support Group include hundreds of former patients and their friends and families (see Appendix). Sometimes the member is a survivor of Prozac, sometimes a friend or relative of someone who became emotionally disturbed, or committed suicide or murder, while on Prozac. McConnell became involved after his fiancée, seemingly out of the blue, strangled her mother to death with a drapery cord. The fiancée was taking Prozac at the time.

The Prozac Survivors Support Group is wholly independent, receives no funding from anyone, and is not affiliated with crank groups or cults. It is run by volunteers.

The survivor group files contain hundreds of cases: The man who thought his cow was leaning to one side and tried to straighten the animal by backing a tractor into it; the woman who thought the roof of her home was dirty and became enraged when her husband didn't appreciate her sitting up there for hours to clean it by hand; ordinary folks who suddenly embezzle or rob banks, and then throw the money away on outlandish schemes.

I have been working closely with the Prozac survivors, addressing their annual conventions, helping them publicize their existence, and benefiting from their moral support and the vast experience reflected in their hundreds of members. I wish more psychiatrists would ask these groups, "What is your data showing?" Our Center for the Study of Psychiatry has published a report that summarizes and evaluates the Prozac survivors' experiences.[12]

I already knew innumerable Prozac horror stories, but I began to meet new survivors and to hear about new tragedies when I appeared on recent TV talk shows. On one show, a brother and sister gave their contrasting views of the drug. The sister had "crashed" and become suicidal after a few weeks of feeling energized on Prozac. More recently her brother had been prescribed Prozac for anxiety related to the Los Angeles earthquake. After a few weeks on the drug, he felt like he was living fully for the first time in his life. He felt more alert, brighter, and happier than ever; but his sister saw ominous personality changes in him, a way of being "out of touch" that mirrored the changes she herself had experienced shortly before she crashed.

On another show, another brother and sister told a far more grim story. Their father, a kind and gentle man who had never been suicidal or aggressive, took Prozac for stress and fatigue. According to his two children, under the drug's influence, without warning or provocation, he stabbed his wife—their mother—to death. After inflicting multiple wounds on her, he killed himself.

In the same week, an attorney called me with yet another sad tale—a woman physician who had prescribed Prozac for herself to combat the stress of starting up a practice and ended up shooting herself. Her husband, a surgeon, was suing Eli Lilly, the manufacturer of Prozac, for failure to warn people about the dangers of the drug. He would have to stand in line behind two dozen or more others who were filing similar suits. Then another attorney called to tell me about a man who had murdered his boss and almost killed his wife while he was taking Prozac.

* * *

Meanwhile, my own clinical experience with Prozac has confirmed the existence of the drug's dark side. As a result of my earlier books, including *Toxic Psychiatry*, and my work as director of the Center for the Study of Psychiatry, I am at times a beacon to people who have been hurt, frustrated, or humiliated by biopsychiatric treatment. Many patients come to me after having failed to improve on a variety of medications. Often they have been damaged by earlier biopsychiatric treatments.

Suffering from chronic neck pain after a skiing accident in Colorado, Gina,* a twenty-seven-year-old woman, had been referred to me by her orthopedist. She had been prescribed a variety of analgesics, and while they helped to relieve her pain, they tended to sap her energy. She'd also been given several different antidepressants, sometimes to ease her physical pain† and at other times to treat her depression. She said, "They just didn't do much for me."

Seven years earlier, Gina had fled from her traditional Sicilian family and come to the United States as a student. She loved her mother and father very much, but chose to reject her father's authoritarian attitudes as well as her mother's and sister's subservience to the males in the family. Gina was simply too spirited—too spontaneously independent—to stand for it.

It was easy for me to believe Gina when she described how she arrived in this country as a student with only a few remote family contacts, learned English in a matter of months, and then demonstrated an unanticipated aptitude for science. She was now a research assistant at a

---

*Unless otherwise indicates, names like Gina's are pseudonyms and the stories have been disguised or even transformed in signfiicant ways in the interest of privacy.

†Some doctors believe that the tricyclic antidepressants, such as Tofranil (imipramine) and Elavil (amitriptyline), can specifically relieve pain. I suspect they mostly dull the emotional response.

rising biotech firm while at the same time getting her master's degree in microbiology.

My psychiatric practice continually confirms the formative influence of childhood in the lives of adults, yet I am regularly astonished at how some people manage to reach adulthood with an intensity of energy and personal courage that seems wholly unexplained in terms of their background. Gina, full of life, was one of them. Out of the bulwark of traditionalism and patriarchy came this brave, self-determined young person. Even while pacing my office in physical pain and emotional despair, Gina emanated spiritual energy.

The skiing accident had occurred eighteen months earlier, leaving Gina with pain and spasms secondary to bruising in the region of her cervical vertebrae. Gina's work in the biotech lab required focusing her eyes through microscopes and calibrating instruments, while turning her head back and forth to make notes or to draw sketches. The effort created tensions in her neck that stymied her recovery. But she resisted taking vacations, let alone sick leave, and so she fought against the pain, tried to keep working, and got worse.

The research chief in Gina's department had singled her out as a rising star and had already included her among the string of more credentialed authors on an upcoming scientific paper. She routinely put in extra hours at the lab and then additional hours going to class and studying. She couldn't let up; she didn't want to let up. She had, in her own words, a "go-go" style. Now, partially disabled by the injury, she was depressed and even suicidal for the first time in her life.

Until the accident, Gina's love life had been as exciting and seemingly ideal as her career. Six years earlier, she had met and soon married Jake, a Jewish-American art dealer. "I was hardly settled down in America," she explained, when she had strolled off the street into an art show at Jake's gallery and, across the crowded room, he'd been drawn by her vibrancy. It began with his offering her a glass of wine and quickly blossomed into a story-book romance. She had worked for a time in his gallery, and then begun school and her eventual career.

Gina described Jake as the most wonderful man imaginable—and promptly began to sob. Their romance had been perfect, or so she thought, until the last year or so. In the beginning, their friends had seen them as the ideal couple. Even her mother and father—to her surprise—overcame the shock of her relationship with a Jewish-American man. After the marriage, they had met and come to accept her warm, vibrant husband. He had capped his trip to Italy by taking them on an art tour of Rome.

Their tradition-oriented families turned out to have much in common, and Gina loved and was loved by Jake's parents. She developed a wide circle of friends, some through school, others through the gallery and work.

"Gone," she told me sadly. "They're all gone."

Six months earlier, she had left her husband and rejected all of her friends. "I was determined," she said, "to do it on my own."

"But your husband—I've never heard a woman speak so lovingly of a man she's determined to divorce."

I don't usually challenge my clients too strongly in the first few sessions of therapy, but her story didn't make emotional sense.

"Gina," I said, "when people are so much in love and have a few years of really good married-time behind them, they don't usually quit so quickly. What was going on?"

"When I made the decision, I felt like I had 'had it with him,' " she said. Then she added, "Besides, I was feeling that way with everyone. I had had it with everyone."

"It still doesn't make sense," I persisted. "He was going through stresses and not faring too well, maybe coming apart, not being himself. And so were you. But the change in your feelings—it sounds so abrupt and final for someone so in love."

"Jake's dad is retired, and he got sick about that time," Gina started to recall the sequence of events. "So Jake went to Palm Springs to help out." It was hard for her to sort out what had happened over these difficult and trying months, and she hadn't pieced this part of the story together. "While Jake was gone—it was a couple of weeks—I got a whole new feeling about being alone. All of a sudden, I felt like I didn't need him or anyone else. I was fine all by myself. Perfect! I began fighting on the phone with my parents. And then I called Jake in California and said I wanted a separation, and he freaked out, and his mom and dad, well they got really angry, and I basically told them all to go to hell."

She stopped as if surveying her life's wreckage for the first time.

"And when my friends said, 'Gina, what are you doing?', I just told them to go to hell, too. Pretty soon, there wasn't anybody."

She stopped for a moment and said, "It doesn't make sense, does it?" Tears were running down her cheeks.

She got up, paced, and then sat back down again, pulling tissues out of the box.

"Gina," I asked, "were you taking any psychiatric medications at the time?"

"Probably."

"Which ones?"

She had to think hard to recall. "A week or two before Jake went away to San Francisco, I got started with a new doctor. He gave me . . . yes. . . . It was Prozac."

During a period of three weeks on Prozac, Gina had rejected everyone in her life.

Any person's life is far too complex to capture in a few paragraphs. Surely many factors, known and unknown, had brought Gina to drive away her friends and relations, and to teeter now on the brink of suicide. But what struck me, and Gina also, was the abruptness of her complete rejection of all the people who loved her and whom she loved as well.

Could Gina's transformation be attributed entirely to Prozac? We can never be certain of this, but starting Prozac coincided with Gina's sudden withdrawal of feeling from family and friends. Ordinarily, it might have seemed like a curiosity, something to be tucked away for future use. But I was recalling something I had already tucked away—a conversation with Ann Tracy, Utah Director of the Prozac Survivors Support Group. It was one of the first things Ann shared with me. She explained, "A lot of what we're seeing is people losing their feeling for the people in their lives. They stop caring about their husbands or wives, or their children. They stop caring about God." Ann knew firsthand. When the man she loved had started taking Prozac, he'd pulled away from her and from everyone else.

The Prozac Craze Perspective

The moral and psychological dangers posed by Prozac are ultimately more threatening than its physical side effects. But this is not the first time that America has fallen unabashedly in love with a *prescription* medication. Until the danger of addiction became obvious, Valium enjoyed an escalating reputation as "mother's little helper." Housewives throughout the country got through their humdrum, frustrating daily chores by remaining in a drug-induced fog. But Valium never benefited from medical and media claims that it improved the normal human condition.[13] The picture is more complicated with the amphetamines, drugs that in many ways resemble Prozac. We shall find that three decades ago, very similar claims were made for their special life-enhancing properties.

While Prozac is not the first prescription drug epidemic, it has garnered a degree of media support never before encountered, as well as a best-selling book by Peter Kramer to fuel its popularity. Kramer bases his theory of Prozac-induced personality transformation on nothing more than a handful of his own cases. He shows a naïve reliance on the manufacturer of Prozac, Eli Lilly, in his discussion of the drug's impact on the brain. In particular, he shows too little awareness of the pharmacological mechanisms that could cause the opposite of Prozac's intended effect, leading patients to become violent or depressed and suicidal. He gives no credence to the Prozac survivor movement.

Kramer argues that Prozac can transform personality for the better but largely dismisses the far more likely possibility that, like any psychoactive drug, it can transform it for the worse. In passing, he makes frequent comparisons of Prozac to amphetamines and cocaine, but ends up superficially rejecting the clinical implications without fully examining the comparisons. He sprinkles his book with moral considerations, but does not seem to take them seriously. While touting the drug's capacity to reduce sensitivity to oneself and others, he fails to face the implications of creating a society of less-in-touch, less-caring, and less-loving human beings. He seems enamored with his concluding observation that "In time, I suspect we will come to discover that modern psychopharmacology has become, like Freud in his day, a whole climate of opinion under which we conduct our different lives."

In my conversations with Kramer and in his media appearances, he seems genuinely concerned that his book has helped to fuel the Prozac craze. He tries, tentatively, to caution the country about moral concerns. On a talk show we appeared on together, he warned that there's no way to anticipate Prozac's potentially damaging effects on the developing brains of children and adolescents. Nevertheless, his book has misled hundreds of thousands of readers and millions more who have heard its message of better living through chemistry.

It's time to address the real issues and questions about Prozac:

- Did Prozac perform well or even adequately during the FDA approval trials, or was the FDA overeager to approve it?
- What are the real adverse effects of Prozac and has the FDA told the public everything it knows?
- What is Prozac's short-term and long-term impact on the brain?
- Is Prozac a clinical and pharmacological cousin to "speed" and cocaine?
- Do some people really function better on Prozac and, if so, what does that mean about their lives?
- Can Prozac encourage or worsen someone's tendency toward violence, depression, and suicide?
- How did Prozac win FDA approval despite its potentially life-threatening behavioral side effects, and why did the agency exonerate the drug at its September 1991 hearing?
- What economic and political forces have backed the promotion of the drug?
- Why is there an avalanche of lawsuits against Eli Lilly regarding Prozac?
- What methods does Lilly use to push America to buy its pill?
- What are the moral and spiritual implications for a nation being flooded by propaganda in favor of taking drugs?
- Are there hidden human costs to taking Prozac that may haunt the individual and end up plaguing society?
- What is depression and what are an individual's alternatives to taking drugs?

America is turning a corner with vast moral, scientific, and medical implications. We may have finally adopted a "National Prescription Drug"—and with it, the idea that drugs are the answer. In less than a generation, we have rejected the motto, "Just say no to drugs," and adopted the motto, "Take this drug to improve your life." It is time for opposing voices. It's time to talk back to Prozac.

TWO

A Primer on How Prozac Is Supposed to Work

WHAT IS PROZAC?

Prozac, and a group of closely related drugs including Zoloft and Paxil, belongs to a new generation of antidepressants that were engineered in drug company laboratories. The drugs are called selective serotonin reuptake inhibitors, or SSRIs. The name provides guideposts for discussing its impact on the brain. We'll begin with serotonin.

Serotonin* is a neurotransmitter—a chemical produced in nerve cells (neurons). Serotonin was discovered in the body and then in the brain in the mid-1950s. Ten years later, in 1964, specific serotonin-containing nerve cells, or neurons, were located in the brain. Further investigations identified serotonin as a neurotransmitter or messenger between brain cells.

A very simplified Diagram A (see page 21) depicts neurotransmission at a serotonergic nerve synapse. Serotonin (labeled as S) is made in the nerve and then released from the nerve ending into a small cleft or space (synapse) between the nerve ending and the next nerve in line.

The serotonergic nerve is called presynaptic because it

*5-Hydroxytryptamine or 5-HT.

DIAGRAM A

Steps Involved in Serotonin Neurotransmission

1. Serotonin (symbolized by "S") is made within the presynaptic nerve, then released into the synapse from the nerve end.
2. Serotonin connects to special receptors on the postsynaptic nerve.
3. Extra serotonin is retaken into the presynaptic nerve end for reuse or destruction.

Prozac blocks reuptake of serotonin. This causes more serotonin to remain in the synapse for a longer time.

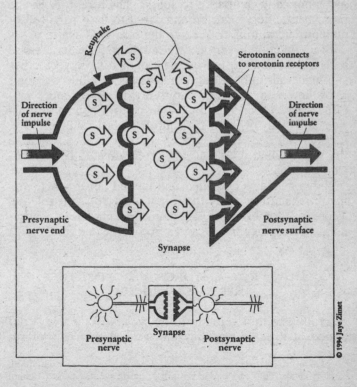

© 1994 Jaye Zimet

deposits the neurotransmitter (in this case, serotonin) into the synapse. The nerve on the other side of the synapse is called postsynaptic, because it receives the neurotransmitter. Serotonin, as it crosses the synapse, acts as the chemical messenger between the two nerves.

After it is released into the synaptic space, the serotonin must connect to special serotonin receivers, called *receptors,* on the surface of the postsynaptic nerve. Once the connection is made, the postsynaptic nerve is fired.

Packets of serotonin, released into the synapse, can be metaphorically compared to sparks. The receptors on the postsynaptic nerve can be compared to flash pans full of gunpowder, waiting to receive the serotonin spark.

Brain function is very complicated and little understood and, in addition to neurotransmitters, a variety of other substances also affect nerve transmission. While we don't know how many neurotransmitters exist, 100 or more substances have been identified that control neurotransmission, and many of them are neurotransmitters. Dopamine, norepinephrine, acetylcholine, and serotonin are among the well-studied ones and are often affected by psychotropic* drugs.

Nerve cells are classified and named according to the neurotransmitter that they manufacture and release. There are, for example, dopaminergic, cholinergic, adrenergic (norepinephrine), and serotonergic nerves.

HOW PROZAC WORKS: BLOCKING THE REUPTAKE PROCESS

Neurotransmitters remain in the synapse for only a brief period of time before they are used, destroyed,† or re-

---

*A psychotropic or psychoactive drug is one that affects the brain, mind, and behavior. The term includes nonpsychiatric agents, such as alcohol or marijuana, as well as prescription medications.

†In the destruction process, serotonin is broken down (degraded or me-

turned to the presynaptic nerve cell for further use. When the neurotransmitter is taken back up by the nerve for reuse, the process is called reuptake, or simply uptake.

Prozac blocks or inhibits the reuptake process for serotonin. The result is an increased amount of serotonin in the synaptic space and a longer duration of action. In effect, more "sparks" are allowed to remain glowing in the synapse. With more serotonin remaining active in the synapse, presumably there will be increased firing of nearby postsynaptic nerves.[1]

Biopsychiatrists theorize that blocking the uptake of serotonin from the synapse increases serotonergic neurotransmission and that this is good for the brain and mind, leading to the improvement of mental disorders, including depression. The theory is based on research and speculations suggesting that sluggish serotonergic nerve transmission is a cause of impulsivity, including violence and suicide. The theory itself is somewhat confusing and contradictory, because it's difficult to conceive of depression as an expression of "impulsivity"; but the theory tries to link together a variety of behaviors or conditions, especially violence, murder, depression, and suicide. Sluggish serotonergic nerve activity is supposed to worsen or cause that entire cluster of destructive tendencies.

Meanwhile, is there evidence that causing serotonergic nerves to become more active can help people to overcome emotional problems? Very little. Almost all the research is about sluggish serotonin, not normal or hyperactive serotonin.

It is presumed that blocking reuptake of a transmitter automatically leads to the "enhancement" of nerve function, but this conclusion seems highly unlikely. It is much

---

tabolized) into 5-Hydroxyindoleacetic acid (5-HIAA). Measurements of the concentration of 5-HIAA in the brain or spinal fluid are often used as rough indicators of the level of serotonergic nerve activity in the brain.

more likely that blocking the normal regulatory activities of the brain would produce widespread *dysfunction*.

THE SUPPOSED SELECTIVITY OF PROZAC

Prozac, Zoloft, and Paxil are described as "selective" uptake blockers. That is, they are supposed to impact on serotonergic nerves with little or no spread of effect to other neurotransmitter systems or other brain functions. This is an important claim because the promotion of Prozac has centered on the concept that, unlike other antidepressants, its effects are relatively limited by virtue of its selective inhibition of serotonin reuptake. In encouraging patients to take the drug, psychiatrists often follow this promotional line, explaining that "Prozac is different. It affects only serotonin." Almost everyone who takes Prozac or any SSRI has heard this.

For many reasons, this claim of selectivity is very misleading. The SSRIs, in fact, end up heavily impacting other neurotransmitter systems. Prozac, for example, has been shown to stimulate indirectly the adrenergic neurotransmitter system, resulting in significant, widespread compensatory changes within the receptors of that system.[2] One of Prozac's most menacing side effects, as we shall see, is probably due at least in part to its effect on yet another neurotransmitter, dopamine.

The emphasis placed on selectivity for the serotonergic system can further mislead people, including physicians, who do not realize that serotonergic nerves spread like a branching tree throughout the brain and spinal cord.

Every neuron is made up of a cell body, dendrites (receptive extensions from the surface of the cell body), and an axon. The axon is a slender filament that reaches out to other neurons and their dendrites and axons to make synapses with them. Some axons are infinitesimally short and some are long enough to extend around much of the brain or down the spinal cord. As depicted in Diagram B

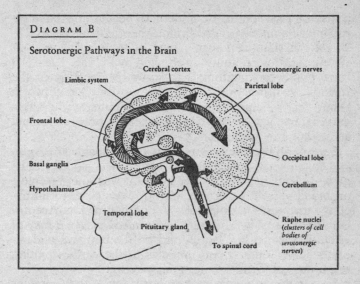

DIAGRAM B

Serotonergic Pathways in the Brain

above, the serotonergic cell bodies lie clumped in the raphe nuclei (a collection of cell bodies) deep in midbrain, but their axons reach into nearly every corner and crevice of the brain and down the spinal cord, where they affect a wide variety of other nerves that control bodily functions. Serotonin is, in fact, the most widespread neurotransmitter system in the brain.[3]

In the process of spreading throughout the brain, serotonin nerves help to regulate every major functional region, including the cerebral cortex, frontal lobes, limbic system, basal ganglia, cerebellum, and hypothalamus. Through the hypothalamus, the system also affects the pituitary gland. Serotonin, therefore, affects many other systems in the brain, including those that produce endorphins, thyroid hormones, corticosteroids (cortisol), and sex hormones.[4]

The serotonin system is the most widespread neurotransmitter system in the brain and, because of this, Prozac impacts on the entire brain. The chart on pages 27–29 lists, in simplified form, some of the central nervous system functions potentially affected by Prozac. The chart corresponds to Diagram B to show the location of the various brain functions within the serotonergic network. While very schematic, the point is accurate: Serotonergic nerves influence the function of the entire brain and mind, and hence the whole person.

Serotonin also plays important roles outside the brain and spinal cord. It was first isolated in the blood, and its name reflects the constrictive action it was found to have on blood vessels. Scientists are not even close to unraveling serotonin's various roles in bodily function. According to a review in the *Pharmacological Basis of Therapeutics,* "5-HT [serotonin] both stimulates and inhibits nerves and smooth muscles in the cardiovascular, respiratory, and gastrointestinal systems."[5]

Prozac has been shown to interfere with the functions of serotonin throughout the body, including the platelets in the blood, accounting in part for its wide variety of side effects.

Overall, Eli Lilly's promotional line about Prozac's selective effects on the nervous system should be viewed with caution and skepticism. No one prescribing or receiving the drug can fully grasp Prozac's overall impact on the brain and whole body, because it's beyond our current scientific understanding.

EFFEXOR: BACK TO THE FUTURE

Now that Prozac, Zoloft, and Paxil have claimed a position of superiority by virtue of selectively impacting on the serotonergic system, we already have a promotional backlash. Effexor (venlafaxine hydrochloride) was approved by the FDA in December 1993 and is now available (spring 1994); it will be marketed as "Prozac with a

Areas of the Brain Affected by the Serotonergic Nerves

Area	Where Located	Effects of Dysfunction
Raphe Nuclei	Deep within the brain	This is the origin for the nerve cells that make and release serotonin. The extensions (axons) of serotonergic nerves spread throughout the brain and into the spinal cord. Prozac and other SSRIs disrupt the function of all serotonergic nerves.
Cerebral Cortex	Outer surface of the brain	Dysfunction within the cerebral cortex impairs higher mental activities, including intelligence and sensory perception.
Frontal Lobes	Front of the brain	Dysfunction within the frontal lobes impairs reason, impulse control, ability to make future plans, empathy and social awareness, insight and judgment—in short, the most human functions.
Limbic System	Widespread, beneath the frontal lobes	Dysfunction within the limbic system affects regulation of emotions, and usually produces indifference and apathy or euphoria.

Areas of the Brain Affected by the Serotonergic Nerves

Area	Where Located	Effects of Dysfunction
Basal Ganglia	Middle of the brain	Dysfunction within the basal ganglia causes abnormal movements, and can cause emotional blunting and mental deterioration.
Temporal Lobes, Including Hippocampus	Lower side and undersurface of the brain	Dysfunction within the temporal lobe impairs the ability to learn and to remember new experiences, and can obliterate old memories.
Parietal Lobe	Toward the back surface of the brain	Dysfunction within the parietal lobe impairs integration and understanding of sensory perceptions, language, and sense of self.
Cerebellum	Lower posterior of the brain	Dysfunction within the cerebellum affects regulation of muscular tone, posture and gait, and coordination, especially of skilled movements.
Hypothalamus	Small area of undersurface of brain above the pituitary gland	Dysfunction within the hypothalamus impairs temperature control, appetite, and hormonal function, including pituitary gland functions.

Areas of the Brain Affected by the Serotonergic Nerves

Area	Where Located	Effects of Dysfunction
Pituitary Gland	Base of the brain	Dysfunction of the pituitary gland can impair thyroid, adrenal, and sexual functions, and can affect overall reaction to stress.
Spinal Cord	Begins at base of brain and extends downward through the vertebral column	Dysfunction within the spinal cord affects nerves that spread throughout the body; especially impaired are reflexes and muscle tone.

NOTE: Each of these functional areas of the brain is labeled on Diagram B (see page 25). This chart gives only a partial review of the various regions of the brain affected by serotonergic neurotransmission.

punch."[6] It blocks the reuptake of not only serotonin but also of norepinephrine.

In bygone days, drug companies bragged about how many neurotransmitters their drugs affected, because all of the neurotransmitter systems were, at one time or another, proposed as participants in the cause of depression. In effect, they had several different punches. Then Prozac outflanked them by making a unique claim for zeroing in on one neurotransmitter system. Now comes Effexor, trying to stake out a special claim for affecting two neurotransmitters.

Although at least eight tricyclic antidepressants are known to block the reuptake of both norepinephrine and serotonin,[7] the manufacturer of Effexor (Wyeth Laboratories Inc.) is claiming greater specificity. In fact, cocaine and amphetamine, like Effexor, block the reuptake of serotonin and norepinephrine. They also block the reuptake of dopamine, so cocaine and amphetamine might be marketed as Prozac with a *double* punch. Soon, I am sure, we will get back to the future with a new antidepressant that boasts of affecting three or more neurotransmitters all at once.

THE SUPPOSED ABILITY OF PROZAC TO CORRECT BIOCHEMICAL IMBALANCES

One of my clients, Harriet, a sensitive and caring young woman who works as a music teacher, had come to me after a brief psychiatric hospitalization during graduate school in which she had been "zonked" by antidepressants and threatened with electroshock. Her former psychiatrist had issued dire warnings about her biochemical imbalance, predicting that without medication for the rest of her life, she would need repeated hospitalizations and electroshock to keep from killing herself. Harriet wanted my help precisely because she did not favor pharmacological approaches, even though she still felt suicidal at the time she came to see me.

Having been orphaned and left with a legacy of shyness, Harriet wanted long-term emotional support and so we worked together for a number of years while she improved her social skills and became more confident at teaching. Eventually, she found the courage to develop an active music teaching practice outside her regular school job.

Despite our best efforts, Harriet still became somewhat depressed during May and June of each year. It was the anniversary of her mother's death and was complicated as well by despondency over the lack of love in her life as springtime approached. We had made a lot of progress—she never became suicidal or required hospitalization, and the periods of despondence grew less intense and briefer—but springtime always brought a temporary gloom into her life.

Then Prozac came out and in May of that year, 1988, Harriet asked me about it. I explained that Prozac did not seem to sedate or subdue people the way some of the older antidepressants did and I gave her some literature and described the various adverse effects. I reassured her that I didn't want to interfere with any of her decisions and when she said she might like to try Prozac, I gave her the name of a well-known and respected biopsychiatrist. She planned to continue seeing me for psychotherapy.

Harriet went to the psychiatrist, who immediately said she had a biochemical imbalance and prescribed Prozac. When she got "hyper" and had trouble sleeping the next week, he added a sedative minor tranquilizer.

The prescribing physician, Harriet told me, seemed very busy, shuffling patients in and out every fifteen minutes, and charging each of them nearly as much as a psychotherapist might for a full hour. When Harriet had trouble getting an evening hour with him, he started filling her prescriptions by telephone. She felt abandoned and asked me to take over the management of the drugs. I agreed and also decided to stop referring patients to my colleague.

Meanwhile, Harriet worked her way through her springtime depression a little more easily than the year before. Neither of us could tell if the drugs had done it, because the springtime depressions had become progressively less troublesome each year. She felt little effect from the two drugs other than a mild constriction of her emotional range.

As the depression lifted, Harriet felt in an emotional bind. She couldn't figure out, in her words, "Did I do it myself or was it the drug?" But that was a minor problem compared to the fear that now overcame her at the thought of stopping either the Prozac or the tranquilizer Klonopin (clonazepam).

Klonopin is habit forming and addictive, and many patients have trouble shaking off the use of one dose at night for sleep. Harriet was convinced the sedative wasn't doing any good because, after all, she fell asleep almost instantly, before it had time to work. But when she tried to stop, she became anxious as night came on. Although I told her she might experience "rebound insomnia"—a hyperactivity of her brain in response to coming off the sedative—she was afraid to wait out the withdrawal period.

Harriet also tried to stop the Prozac, and although her depression didn't come back in the few days she was off it, she again became too frightened to discontinue the drug. Occasionally I reminded her about the problems associated with long-term drug use, but, as of now, she has been unable to stop taking either one. Yet she still worries about long-term adverse effects and so do I. The drugs are definitely producing biochemical imbalances.

Whenever I give a public talk, someone is bound to confront me on the subject of biochemical imbalances. I'll be told in no uncertain terms, "My doctor says I have a biochemical imbalance and I *know* I do!" or "Prozac corrected my biochemical imbalance. It was genetic."

Ever since antidepressants were discovered, it has been assumed that they work because of their effect on nerve transmission in the brain. It has also been assumed that, because they work, there must be something wrong with the nerves they affect. This assumption is commonly used as the major reason for searching for a biochemical cause of depression and other psychiatric disorders. It goes like this: The drugs work, the drugs affect the brain, so there must be something wrong with the brain. But this is faulty and unscientific reasoning. Many well-known drugs, such as caffeine and alcohol, affect the mind and brain in the absence of any underlying defect in the brain.

The biochemical imbalance theory has replaced Freud's psychological theory as the most widely accepted explanation for emotional pain and suffering. Freud's theory in turn had replaced more religious and philosophical explanations, such as original sin, the devil, and moral degeneracy. The modern biopsychiatric theory, however, does have one thing in common with Freud's unconscious—both can be misused to make people dependent on mental health experts to explain what's really going on inside them.

Freud's psychological theories have some validity and usefulness. Mental processes are influenced by childhood experiences that the individual cannot recall and by feelings and attitudes that lie outside awareness. A person can take better control of his or her own life by becoming more self-aware. The unconscious, in this sense, does describe a real aspect of human experience and can be a helpful, empowering concept.

The mind and behavior are also affected by dysfunctions in the brain, such as Alzheimer's disease. Hormonal imbalances produced by disorders like hyper- or hypothyroidism can affect mood.* The known biochemical im-

---

*Estrogen and, in case of hysterectomies or tubal ligations, testosterone,

balances produced by psychiatric medications, as well as by other drugs, frequently cause severe emotional disturbances. But this does not mean that a significant percentage of people who seek psychiatric help have anything physically wrong with their brains.

There is, in fact, very little evidence that they do. If depression, for example, has a biological or genetic basis, it has not been demonstrated scientifically. To the contrary, each new biological hypothesis ends up discredited. Biopsychiatric theory remains pure speculation and runs counter to a great deal of research and clinical experience, as well as common sense.*

Even if emotional suffering turns out to be caused at times by subtle biochemical imbalances, can these physical problems be corrected by currently available psychiatric drugs? Or would the drugs make matters worse by adding more gross biochemical imbalances to the existing disorder? The following case history illustrates the problem.

Mike Donnelly was one of those who traveled far to present his concerns at the 1991 FDA hearing on Prozac. The chemical-imbalance theory confused him into believing he was "crazy," when he was, instead, having an adverse reaction to Prozac. Mike testified:

---

can drop below an optimum level causing fatigue, clouded thinking, sleep disturbances and other phenomena easily mistaken for depression. John Arpels, M.D., associate clinical professor of obstetrics and gyneoclogy at the University of California, San Francisco, confirmed this in a recent interview with us (also see Laurence, 1994). Arpels has worked with women who felt the need to take Prozac or other SSRIs until they received hormone replacement therapy. Too often the possibility of low sex hormone levels is not explored before a patient is started on antidepressants. Arpel believes that the clinical manifestations of sex hormone deficiency can sometimes be more reliable than blood levels.

*Biological and genetic theories of psychiatric disorders are critically evaluated in my book, *Toxic Psychiatry* (1991). I explore the psychosocial viewpoint in that book and in *Beyond Conflict* (1992). We will also return to these questions throughout this book.

I am Mike Donnelly. It is a matter of moral responsibility that I am here today. I'm a successful business- and family man from south Florida. I'm a Christian and do not belong to the Church of Scientology.* I've always been mentally healthy and well blessed.

Two years ago I sustained a massive head injury due to a car accident. After months of treatment and rehabilitation I tried to go back to work and run my business. I became frustrated by my inability to function as I used to. My doctor recommended I see a psychiatrist to help me through this anxiety.

I met with this psychiatrist and he had me fill out these mental test forms in which one question asked if I had thoughts of killing myself. Well, this question shocked me and I checked no. It went on to ask several more questions. I filled them all out. He then graded these tests and gave me a high score on them, what you would call, perhaps, an A on my mental condition at the time.

He then declared, through no scientific test, that I had a chemical imbalance in my brain due to the head trauma and which could be corrected by taking America's new wonder drug, Prozac, and showed me *Newsweek* magazine proclaiming this statement on the cover. . . .

The first week taking Prozac I felt no effects. The second week my anxiety increased, I could not make decisions, and I had trouble eating and sleeping. The third week I became agitated and could not sit still. I began pacing through my house and had more trouble eating and sleeping. The fourth week I had total loss of appetite, complete insomnia, anxiety was literally pouring out of my ears. After not sleeping or eating the entire week, I was incapable of any rational thinking and reduced to a pa-

---

*To deflect criticism, Eli Lilly and its supporters have purposefully tried to attribute the widespread public and professional concern over Prozac exclusively to the Church of Scientology. While the Church of Scientology has been active in publicizing the dangers of Prozac, it is by no means alone in doing so. Our Center for the Study of Psychiatry, for example, has no affiliation with Scientology and does not work with the group in any capacity. The various psychiatric survivor groups, including the Prozac Survivors Support Group (see Appendix), are also unrelated to the Church of Scientology.

thetic shell of a person with nothing inside. I felt like I literally lost my soul, incapable of any emotion whatsoever.

At this time I did not attribute these effects to Prozac but merely saw my head trauma from the car accident was getting worse. My anxiety became humanly intolerable and I became convinced I was never going to be the same, that the only way to have peace and serenity again was to die. This is how I became intensely suicidal.

I would like to describe "intensely suicidal" for you. I wanted to throw myself under our large company dump trucks as they were pulling out for work. I fantasized about drinking weedkiller, throwing myself on high-voltage power lines, running across a police practice gun range in full fire, wrestling a gun from a policeman's belt while in a crowded store, jumping off the balcony of my parent's 10th-floor condominium, and many more suicide fantasies.

I realized I needed help at this point and went back to the psychiatrist, who recommended I double my dose of Prozac. I [agreed to commit] myself to an institution, where I would be safe and could be properly monitored. After visiting two institutions, with my bags packed, ready to commit myself, I lay down on the bed in a room that would have been mine. I remember staring up and looking at the ceiling for several minutes. Then I got up, I walked over to my wife and I said, "I can't do this, I'm leaving."

I walked out the door and got in the car and left, as a passenger—I couldn't even drive a car. On the way home my wife yelled at me and said I had to listen to the doctors, I had to stay in the hospital, and I did not even want to help myself. On the way home I got a glimmer of what might be happening to me, and when I returned home I walked straight into my bathroom, opened up my medicine cabinet and took out the bottle of Prozac and said, "This stuff is killing me," and flushed it down the toilet.

This was after two months of taking it. I said, "I'm not taking this drug anymore, seeing a psychiatrist or committing myself to an institution. Instead I'll take vitamins and start working out." Then I barged out my front door and made a feeble attempt at jogging around the block.

For the next month and a half this nightmare raged on. I still had insomnia, high anxiety, and suicidal thoughts and was not sure it was definitely Prozac causing this. Little by little my anxiety subsided. I began sleeping again and suicidal thoughts subsided.

Once again I was capable of rational thinking. I read some literature about the tremendous adverse reactions that can be caused by Prozac and it was like reading about what I had just gone through. I realized that this was Prozac that had pushed me to the brink of self-destruction and I could be normal again. . . .

In retrospect, Mike no longer believes that he had a biochemical imbalance. In his testimony, he said:

I have found psychiatrists abuse this generalized statement of a chemical imbalance of the brain as a way to prescribe these psychiatric drugs and a way to start the psychiatric revolving door, just go in and out, in and out, and sometimes the problem is you never come out.

Curiously, in light of so much psychiatric concern about the dangers of biochemical imbalances, all known psychiatric drugs produce widespread chemical imbalances in the brain, usually involving multiple systems of nerves. Prozac is no exception.

Many psychoactive substances produce profound effects on people who have nothing wrong with their brains. In fact, in sufficiently large doses all the commonly used psychoactive drugs seem to affect all people without exception. This is also true of all the routinely used street drugs, from marijuana to cocaine. It is true of caffeine, nicotine, and alcohol. Taking into account normal biological variation in responses to drugs, these agents affect everyone in about the same way. Some people like the effects more than others, and believe that the particular drug is beneficial, but there's no reason to believe that they are reacting in a unique fashion. It doesn't take a "broken brain" to respond to drugs; it just takes a brain.

Patients taking Prozac may react in a variety of ways that seem positive or negative to them. Any psychoactive drug—one that affects the brain and mind—is likely to have very different effects on different people. Some people seem to imbibe relatively large quantities of alcohol with seemingly little intoxication, while others take a few sips and become woozy and lose their coordination. Some people can have an occasional social drink, while for others a taste is a prelude to a binge. Some people abuse alcohol for years with seemingly little negative effect, while others develop physical and psychological problems within a short time. Some people become more passive "under the influence" and others more aggressive. Some people hate alcohol and some people love it.

Many people use alcohol regularly "to get through the day." They find it gives them the "courage" to go on. In effect, alcohol is their self-administered medication. Others, seeing the habit in a less favorable light, call it "maintenance drinking," a form of chronic alcoholism.

We should expect to find this wide range of responses to any psychoactive drug, including the SSRIs such as Prozac, Zoloft, and Paxil, as they disrupt the normal brain processes of the individual. That psychiatric drugs have their effect by impinging on normal brain processes is now being demonstrated in the widespread use of Prozac. People with no obvious psychiatric disorder are claiming to benefit from it.

As I describe in detail in *Toxic Psychiatry* (1991), the neurotransmitter theory remains wholly unproven in regard to any psychological or psychiatric disorder. It's pure speculation. Even advocates of the theory point out that the picture is much too complicated to finger one neurotransmitter as the cause of depression. At a recent program sponsored by the Association for Research in Nervous and Mental Diseases, John Krystal of the Yale University School of Medicine declared, "Depression is much more complex than we would have thought not long ago. It is premature to rule out the involvement of any neurotransmitter system." Krystal went on to say it was "naïve" to point to one neurotransmitter, such as serotonin, as the cause of depression. He observed that antidepressant action clearly involved more than a simple increase in the availability of one neurotransmitter.[8]

In fact, it's also premature to assume that abnormalities in *any* neurotransmitter systems, including a combination of them, play any role in depression. The biochemical-imbalance theory is merely the latest biopsychiatric speculation, presented to the public as a scientific truth. And it's the theory behind Prozac. It's thought that by blocking the reuptake of serotonin out of the synaptic space, sluggish nerve transmission is transformed into normal nerve transmission.

The ironic truth is this: The only known biochemical imbalances in the brains of nearly all psychiatric patients are those caused by the treatments. Those rare exceptions who have *known* hormonal disorders, such as Graves' disease (hyperthyroidism) or Cushing's syndrome (adrenocortical hormone excess), are almost always treated as medical rather than psychiatric patients.

CLEVERNESS IS NOT WISDOM

There are more cells in each of our individual brains than there are stars in the sky. The brain is made up of several hundred billion neurons and trillions of synapses. Each individual human brain is more complex than the entire physical universe with all its stars and planets, and with all the various forces, such as gravity, that are at work in it. Unlike the physical universe, the biochemical activities that run the brain remain almost wholly shrouded in mystery. We have no idea, for example, how the brain makes a thought or an emotion. It seems foolhardy to imagine that blocking one of the brain's biochemical functions would somehow improve the brain and mind.[9]

As technologically advanced as the manufacture of Prozac may seem, it does not reflect an equal depth of understanding about how the brain and mind function. At the root lies a dangerous assumption that it is safe and effective to tamper with the most complex organ in the universe. With that in mind, we turn to examining the efficacy and safety of the SSRIs.

THREE

The Real Story Behind Prozac's Approval by the FDA

Most people seem to believe that the FDA conducts its own independent studies of drugs and then decides whether or not to approve them. Nothing could be further from the truth. The FDA, in fact, doesn't have any money to perform its own studies during the approval process for drugs.

All FDA drug studies are constructed, supervised, and paid for by the drug companies themselves, using doctors and research teams of their own choosing—often people with long-established relationships with the company. It seems obvious, but should be underscored, that the pharmaceutical companies do everything they can to make their studies turn out right.

How the Prozac Studies Were Constructed

Regulations require that a new drug must prove its efficacy in double-blind controlled studies comparing it to placebo and to other drugs of established efficacy. Double-blind means that neither the doctors nor the patients know who is getting what kind of pill. Placebo-controlled means that some patients in a comparison control group will be given an inactive substance in pill form—the placebo, or sugar pill. The placebo is, in effect, a fake drug.

If, for example, Prozac does not perform any better than the placebo, Prozac will be seen as ineffective.

Placebo plays a key role in scientific drug studies because it's been repeatedly demonstrated that up to 50 percent or more of depressed patients improve on the sugar pill.[1] In some studies, nearly 90 percent have improved on placebo.

The FDA allowed Lilly to use the "placebo washout," a very questionable but commonly used technique in drug studies.[2] All patients were started off on placebo for approximately one week (4–14 days). Those patients who showed improvement on placebo were then dropped from the study and the trials were begun all over again from scratch with a placebo and a drug group.[3]

Using the placebo washout helps make a drug seem more effective than it is. For example, some of those patients "washed out" of the testing because they responded positively to the placebo might *not* have reacted positively to the drug if they had received it in the second part of the testing. That is, if they had not been dropped from the actual trials, the placebo responders might have once again reacted positively to the sugar pill but not to the drug with its frequently unpleasant side effects. Even if the placebo washout reduced the number of positive responders equally in both the sugar pill and the drug groups, this reduction in the total number of positive responders in both groups would favor the drug. Why? Statistically, the same difference between two smaller groups is more significant than the same difference between two larger groups. The placebo washout purposely produces an unnatural pool of patients. It is unscientific.

Before the FDA approves a psychiatric drug, it typically requires that the drug company produce two or more research protocols that demonstrate significant efficacy for the drug. Each protocol has a specific set of rules developed by the drug company. In the case of Prozac, one protocol included ten separate studies under different leadership at different sites.

The results were then pooled to make one pool of data for statistical purposes. The total number of individual studies or research projects in the various Prozac protocols varied from one to ten.

A typical Lilly protocol for Prozac in its FDA approval process required randomly dividing a group of depressed patients into two similar sections. One section was given placebo for four to six weeks and the other was given Prozac for the same period of time. In other protocols, the group was divided into three parts: one taking placebo; one taking Prozac; and one taking an older, proven antidepressant for comparison.

The protocols used a variety of tests to evaluate week-by-week improvement. Some of these involved self-assessment, but most entailed brief interviews with professionals who checked off symptoms lists. No intensive interviews were utilized.

Each individual study was directed by a principle investigator, a psychiatrist selected by Eli Lilly to ensure that the project was conducted according to the principles laid down by the drug company. Some studies were carried out at universities and others at private research firms that specialize in performing drug company sponsored research.

How the Subjects Were Selected

Potential subjects were interviewed by investigators in each study to determine whether or not they met the standards for major depression as defined in the American Psychiatric Association's *Diagnostic and Statistical Manual of Mental Disorders, Third Edition, Revised (DSM-III-R).** To qualify for major depression, the individual must show signs of depressed mood or loss of pleasure or in-

*In the final chapter we will look in greater depth at the question "What is depression?"

terest in life. These are the first two items on a list of nine items, and the individual must suffer from at least a total of five. The other criteria include the following: significant weight change; sleep disturbance; psychological and physical agitation or retardation; fatigue or loss of energy nearly every day; feelings of worthlessness or "excessive or inappropriate guilt"; indecisiveness and other signs of difficulty thinking and concentrating; and recurrent thoughts of death or suicide.

Most people believe that when Prozac was approved for depression, it had been thoroughly tried on extremely depressed patients and had proven life-saving.

In actuality, the Prozac studies as designed by Lilly excluded all patients with serious tendencies toward suicide. This deliberate exclusion was part of the formal protocol, or organization, of each study used for FDA approval in the United States.* Advocates of the drug would wholly overlook this in their enthusiastic reviews, giving the false impression that Prozac is a potentially life-saving drug. No antidepressant has ever been shown to prevent suicide, and Eli Lilly apparently didn't want to risk finding out whether Prozac would also fail to prevent suicide.

Hospitalized psychiatric patients were also excluded from nearly all of the studies, including every one that was used to approve the drug.

There were no children or elderly adults in the Lilly sponsored FDA studies of Prozac. Once any drug is approved for marketing by the FDA, however, there is nothing to stop psychiatrists from prescribing it for these vulnerable groups. Prozac, in fact, is being widely recommended for children and youth. One such recommendation is in a recent popular book by Columbia University professor of psychiatry Ronald Fieve.[4] Fieve states, "although scientific research in this area is scanty and incomplete the evidence so far indicates that children and

*For the exclusion of "serious suicide risk" patients, see Food and Drug Administration, October 3, 1988, pp. 19, 21, and 23.

adolescents can safely be given Prozac. . . ." The potentially tragic consequences of this practice are underscored in the findings of the government's General Accounting Office (GAO) investigation of the FDA—that children are especially likely to fall victim to adverse reactions that slip through the FDA premarketing tests of drugs.

HOW LARGE AND HOW LONG WERE THE STUDIES

Misleading totals for patients tested in clinical trials are common. In *Everything You Need to Know About Prozac* (1991), psychiatrist Jeffrey Jonas from Fair Oaks Hospital in Summit, New Jersey,* and medical writer Ron Schaumburg defended Prozac by stating, "Some of the reassurance comes from the data on over 11,000 patients who took the drug in clinical trials."

The 11,000 figure appears in an August 31, 1990, "Dear Doctor" letter written by Eli Lilly to American physicians to counteract concerns that Prozac could increase suicidality. The letter states, "More than 11,000 individuals participated in clinical trials for Prozac, including over 6,000 treated with Prozac." Jonas and Schaumburg must have misread this statement, since it indicates that the drug was actually taken by "over 6,000" patients rather than 11,000 patients. However, when a drug company bandies about large—if relatively meaningless—numbers, the numbers are likely to be misread or misinterpreted in favor of the company. The figure of 6,000 patients, meanwhile, is itself potentially misleading.

The drug label as reprinted in the *Physicians' Desk Reference (PDR)* states that there were "5,600 Prozac-exposed" individuals in the premarketing period of

---

*Now a full-time employee of the Upjohn Company, the maker of the psychiatric drugs Xanax and Halcion.

evaluation.* But this apparently includes patients given the drug under a variety of conditions other than actual clinical trials. In another place in the *PDR,* it is stated that 4,000 patients received Prozac in "US premarketing clinical trials." But most of these patients, apparently, were not in placebo-controlled studies—the only ones relevant for efficacy studies. A table of adverse reactions in the *PDR* reviews 1,730 patients who were involved in "placebo-controlled clinical trials."

When we focus on the actual numbers of patients in the trials used by the FDA in the drug approval process, the totals shrink much further. Only three favorable protocols, involving seventeen studies and several hundred patients, were found scientifically adequate enough by the FDA to use them as evidence for approving the drug. Using material obtained through the Freedom of Information Act, I went through each of these seventeen studies, one by one, to add up *the number of Prozac patients who actually completed the four-, five-, or six-week trials* used as the basis for FDA approval. The grand total turned out to be a meager 286 patients.

It is astonishing to realize that the approval of Prozac was based on fewer than 300 patients culled, by various means that we will examine, from the original cast of thousands. It is safe to guess that few if any physicians or patients who rely on FDA studies have any idea that the actual number of Prozac patients completing the trials was so small.

Most people imagine that patients in the FDA approval studies take the test drugs for months and years on end before the drug can be approved, but as we've already pointed out, the scientifically controlled trials for Prozac lasted only a few weeks. An occasional less scientifically rigorous project lasted longer, but 86 percent of all the patients in all the studies were treated for "three months

*An October 3, 1988, Food and Drug Administration report states that 6,070 were exposed to Prozac in U.S. studies, and 1,850 abroad (p. 27).

or less." *Only 63 patients were on fluoxetine for a period of more than two years before completion of the premarketing studies and the FDA approval of Prozac.*[5] In effect, anyone now taking Prozac for more than a few weeks is part of a giant ongoing experiment on its longer-term effects. ·

Failures Are Forgiven

According to the FDA approval process, it doesn't matter how many times a drug *fails* to prove useful in its clinical trials. Innumerable scientific studies can show the drug to be ineffective, but as long as two or more show statistical superiority over placebo, the drug can win approval.

In its "Summary of Basis of Approval," dated October 3, 1988,[6] the FDA states that fourteen protocols involving controlled studies were submitted by Lilly. Four compared Prozac to placebo, and of these, three were used by the FDA as evidence of some beneficial effect. One showed none at all. Of the remaining ten studies, eight showed Prozac to have no positive effect. Overall, there were more negative efforts than positive, but this made no difference in the approval process.

In six out of the seven studies where it was included, imipramine (Tofranil), a very old drug, did better than Prozac.[7] That, too, made no difference in the approval process.

These results do not sound very inspiring, but an examination of the three positive protocols will prove much more disheartening. The analysis that follows was painstakingly garnered from several volumes of FDA data that were decidedly not user-friendly. It is worth giving the reader this rare, and perhaps unprecedented, window into the FDA—a seldom illuminated region of the government.

Protocol 27: Scrambling to Make It

One of the three sets of protocols used to prove the efficacy of Prozac was called Protocol 27. The following information about the protocol is taken from the Food and Drug Administration's March 28, 1985, "Review and Evaluation of Efficacy Data." All page numbers refer to that document.

At the start, Protocol 27 involved more than 700 patients at six separate sites in studies run by different principal investigators. But by the time the entire protocol was completed, and all the data from one of the six sites was excluded, fewer than 150 Prozac patients remained in the whole protocol. Of these, only 104 completed the six-week trials.

The protocol compared three agents: Prozac; an older antidepressant called imipramine (Tofranil); and placebo. The six separate studies, as reported by the drug company and then further analyzed and summarized by the FDA, produced the following results:

1. J. P. Feighner, M.D., from the Feighner Institute in San Diego, according to the FDA found that the older antidepressant, Tofranil, showed significant improvement in the patients in "all variables." However, "fluoxetine was not shown to be consistently different than placebo" (p. 21). In other words, Prozac was a bust.

   An April 3, 1984, in-house FDA memo by Walter Sloboda, a psychologist in the Division of Scientific Investigation, discussed criticisms of Feighner's studies based on an on-site FDA investigation. Among other things, the FDA found that in Protocol 27 a patient was mistakenly given Prozac in addition to Tofranil and that the error had not been properly recorded. Also, in several cases, a variety of abnormal laboratory findings were ignored, entailing risk to patients. Dr. Feighner, the report said, agreed with these observations by the FDA and promised to remedy them.

In addition, Sloboda's memo discussed a consumer complaint in which a patient alleged that she had been given Prozac in a trial and that this initiated an emotional deterioration resulting in hospitalization and electroshock treatment. We have no information on the outcome of the investigation concerning the patient's complaint.

Feighner's practices in conducting Prozac research were criticized again in an August 7, 1984, letter from the FDA's Frances O. Kelsey, Ph.D., M.D., Director of the Division of Scientific Investigation, Office of Compliance, Center for Drugs and Biologics. Kelsey found that Feighner "had several departures from Food and Drug Administration regulations or commonly accepted drug investigational practices." Without mentioning specific deviations, the letter emphasized the need for Feighner to follow the inclusion and exclusion criteria of the studies.*

2. Jay B. Cohn, M.D., a psychiatrist from the University of California in Los Angeles, produced according to the FDA report "seemingly overwhelmingly positive results." However, the statistical manipulations required to achieve them were scientifically unacceptable. For example, Cohn ended up comparing how the Prozac patients did at six weeks with how the placebo patients did at two weeks. Reluctant to come down too hard on a drug company, the FDA observed, "Hence, this study can, at best, be said to be supportive" (p. 27). In contrast to patients on Prozac, patients on the older antidepressant did show im-

---

*Feighner was also involved in Protocol 62 (page 58) and it was unclear whether one or both Prozac protocols were involved in some of these criticisms.

provement. Another Prozac bust.

Cohn, meanwhile, had been sent an extraordinarily critical letter from Frances O. Kelsey, Ph.D., M.D., Director, Division of Scientific Investigations of the FDA. The inspection under the FDA's Bioresearch Monitoring Program found that Cohn had failed to indicate that two of the subjects suffered from a "past history of alcoholism" and that a third subject, who had been treated three times for alcoholism in the prior year, had cirrhosis of the liver. It was also found that in an earlier study in the Prozac FDA approval process, Cohn had failed to obtain written informed consent and had "backdated the consent form."

Eventually the FDA discarded the Cohn study as invalid. Nonetheless, in 1985 Cohn and Charles Wilcox, M.B.A., published the study in the *Journal of Clinical Psychiatry* as part of an Eli Lilly sponsored symposium. They describe their study as an unambiguous success story for Prozac. They give no recognition of the fact that the FDA invalidated and rejected this study. As far as the general medical community knows to this very day, the Cohn study unequivocally proved the efficacy of Prozac.

3. David L. Dunner, M.D., a psychiatrist from the University of Washington in Seattle, found the older antidepressant was effective. But according to the FDA, "There was essentially no difference in efficacy between fluoxetine and placebo" (p. 34). A third failure for Prozac.

4. Bernard I. Grosser, M.D., from the department of psychiatry of the University of Utah, came up with the same negative result as Dunner. According to the FDA, "imipramine produced significantly more improvement than placebo on all major efficacy variables at endpoint." However, fluoxetine was not shown to be consistently different than placebo (p. 42). A fourth negative outcome for Prozac.

Grosser's seeming bias in favor of Prozac is disclosed in an October 26, 1984, letter of complaint sent to him by FDA official Frances Kelsey. Among other criticisms, Kelsey observed that Grosser's informed consent form did not conform with regulations because it describes Prozac ". . . as effective or more effective than imipramine. . . ." Kelsey explained, "Since the purpose of the investigational drug studies is to prove the drug's safety and effectiveness, such statements cannot be made while the drug is being evaluated." Interestingly, Grosser's study failed to confirm his bias.

5. F. S. Abuzzahab, Sr., M.D., from the University of Minnesota Department of Psychiatry, again according to the FDA's analysis, showed that Prozac "produced more improvement than placebo on a few variables. The differences, however, were not consistent and included only some key variables" (p. 47). The older antidepressant was no better. This was essentially a fifth bust.

A December 13, 1984, letter from the FDA's Frances Kelsey to Abuzzahab was critical of his practices in Lilly–sponsored Prozac studies. The letter stated, "Objectionable conditions were found to exist in both of the clinical studies for most of the subjects audited." In particular, the inspection found "that you did not adhere to the protocols and that you did not give proper notification" when making protocol changes.

6. James D. Bremner, M.D., a psychiatrist in Olympia, Washington, did find that Prozac, like the older antidepressant, was better than placebo on "most variables," according to the FDA. This was the only positive study among the six for Prozac. The older antidepressant, however, seemed more effective than Prozac, showing improvement on all variables (p. 30). Only 22 patients finished on Prozac. As another important confounding factor, about one-third of the patients received other psychiatric medications—mi-

nor tranquilizers and sedatives—in addition to Prozac. There is no way to tell if the results would have been positive if the patients had taken Prozac by itself.

In addition to these individual problems with the studies in Protocol 27 that we have mentioned, all of the protocols came under severe criticism. The FDA's November 13, 1984, "In-House Meeting on Fluoxetine" brought together the leading agency officials concerned with monitoring the Prozac application process, including the division head, Paul Leber. The minutes of the meeting, written by Tony De Cicco, stated, "This Agency has discovered a flaw in the experimental design and execution of the Fluoxetine studies." The flaw was located in "the main efficacy trials," seemingly indicating all the studies we will be examining in this chapter.

According to De Cicco's minutes, patients who were not doing well after the second week of the efficacy studies had the double-blind broken and, if found to be taking placebo or Tofranil, were then switched to Prozac. The blind was then broken at six weeks in patients doing well, in order to continue them on their assigned medication after the study.

The manipulations caused two extreme compromises of all the studies. First, as indicated in the analysis of the Cohn study, the efficacy of Prozac at six weeks ended up being compared to the efficacy of placebo at two weeks— a very "biased" analysis. Second, with the blind broken, investigator bias could compromise the results.

In addition, the "In-House Meeting on Fluoxetine" found that very large dropout rates were impairing the analysis of data. The minutes were especially critical of the seemingly positive results of the Cohn study, but the criticism also applied to all the individual studies in all the main efficacy protocols.

The problems found in these efficacy studies should

have invalidated them. But Lilly was allowed to present its data for approval by the FDA.

Despite the bias in favor of Prozac built into the studies by Lilly, at the conclusion of Protocol 27 the picture looked very grim for the drug. But Lilly did not give up. It reshuffled the data, first by removing some but not all of Cohn's embarrassing data. Then Lilly excluded all patients who had received other psychiatric medications along with Prozac. Finally, it *pooled* the pruned data from the remaining five studies into one batch for statistical analysis, treating them as if they belonged to one study. This increased the total number of subjects for analysis, making it easier to demonstrate statistical significance for relatively minor improvements in the Prozac patients.

According to the FDA's March 28, 1985, efficacy review, the results of this strained effort to pool the data were not convincing: "Imipramine was clearly more effective than placebo, whereas fluoxetine was less consistently better than placebo." The FDA concluded, "This study is supportive but not strongly positive in demonstrating fluoxetine's role in the treatment of depression" (p. 49). Basically, Prozac had been shown, once again, to be a bust.

Undaunted, Lilly reworked the numbers one more time and resubmitted the new calculations to the FDA, now excluding all of the Cohn data as invalid, and again pooling the other five sites. Discarding the Cohn study eliminated 25 percent of the total protocol patients who completed the six-week trials and should have rendered the pooling process invalid; but the FDA accepted it. At the FDA's request, Lilly also reincluded all the patients who had been given additional psychiatric drugs during their Prozac trials. And at last, pay dirt. Lilly managed to come up with a positive result for the pooled studies on four of several measurements of improvement. Based entirely on the reworked figures, and ignoring the multiple flaws and the failure of all but one of the individual studies to demonstrate efficacy, the FDA concluded: "The re-

vised pooling of Protocol 27 can be said to contribute to
the judgment of substantial evidence of efficacy" (p. 50-
A).

Pooling data from separate *negative* studies in order to
get a *positive* overall result is open to criticism. In fact,
the FDA's own regulations on advertising specifically reject the use of such manipulations. The regulations state
that drug company ads should *not* "use statistics based on
pooled data from inconclusive studies."[8] These particular
pooled studies were worse than "inconclusive"; all but
one were outright negative.

Pooling negative studies is questionable enough. Dropping one of the studies in the process, eliminating 25 percent of the Prozac patients who completed the trials, is
wholly unacceptable.

Notice the extremes to which Lilly and the FDA had
to go to make the numbers work. Notice how much this
has to do with statistical juggling and how little with real
people. There's no indication that any person actually re-
covered from major depression, because *that wasn't even
addressed.* Instead, they were tested for relative degrees
of improvement compared to the placebo patients as
measured on symptom checklists. Although patients had
to meet the *DSM-III-R* criteria for major depression in
order to be admitted into the study, the patients were not
reinterviewed at the conclusion to see if they had recov-
ered and no longer warranted the diagnosis.

There is evidence that the patients themselves did *not*
feel dramatically improved on Prozac. Of the two rating
scales that allowed the patients to record their own impression of the drug, one showed no difference between
Prozac and placebo, and one showed some efficacy for
the drug.

Could the clinicians have been influenced in their positive judgments of Prozac even though they were not supposed to know which patients were getting the drug? Yes.
Prozac patients, as we shall see, have characteristic side
effects—such as insomnia, nightmares, anxiety and ner-

vousness, upset stomach, and weight loss—that could have allowed the rating physicians to guess who was on what drug. In particular, the other drug in the study, Tofranil (imipramine), is very sedating, while Prozac is activating. Consciously or unconsciously, accurately guessing who was on the drug could have influenced the ratings by the doctors.

Earlier we pointed out that studies that fail are forgiven. There's another way this forgiveness takes place *within* each and every study. Overall in Protocol 27, only slightly more than one-half of the Prozac patients managed to stay on the drug for the whole six weeks. The others dropped out, usually because of adverse drug effects and lack of efficacy. How is it possible to claim, as many psychiatrists have, that 70 to 80 percent of patients benefit from Prozac, when as much as 50 percent of the patients do not even continue taking the drug for a brief six-week trial?

The high dropout rate in these six-week-long studies in part answers a frequently asked question, "Why are the drug studies so short?" In the case of Prozac, if the studies had been even a week or two longer, the trend indicates that the vast majority of the Prozac patients would have dropped out, underscoring the failure of the drug as a therapeutic agent.

In summary, in a multisite protocol in which only one of six studies turned out positive for Prozac, pooled data were shuffled and reshuffled, with much of it eliminated, in order to reach statistical significance on a few measures. These machinations were essentially flawed from the start by conditions such as the placebo washout, the extremely short length of the trials, the very small numbers of Prozac patients who completed the trials, the use of superficial symptom checklists to determine efficacy, the exclusion of suicidal or hospitalized patients, the inclusion of patients on multiple psychiatric drugs, and the better performance of the older antidepressant.

Interestingly, Lilly employees Paul Stark, Ph.D., and C. David Hardison, Ph.D., published the results of the pooled data from the five studies without mentioning the fact that the individual studies failed to show efficacy for Prozac, without mentioning the various FDA criticisms, and without giving the impression that Prozac's performance was at best weak. Unlike the FDA analysis and conclusion, which shows Tofranil to be superior to Prozac, the Lilly version claims Prozac to be as effective as ("comparable to") Tofranil.

Protocol 19: More Doubts

Another of the three key positive Prozac protocols, Protocol 19, was conducted by Louis Fabre, Jr., a Houston, Texas, psychiatrist who frequently does FDA research on behalf of drug companies. According to the FDA's March 28, 1985, review, the placebo washout was again employed, and "serious suicidal risk" was an excluding factor (p. 52). Fabre compared Prozac and placebo. Only 47 patients were entered into the study, 10 were then dropped because they couldn't be properly evaluated, and ultimately only 25 finished the trials. *Of these completers, only 11 had been given Prozac* (p. 58).

With this slim number of patients completing the protocol, obtaining a positive result involved considerable statistical maneuvering. For example, an additional five Prozac and seven placebo patients were counted in the statistical analysis for efficacy, even though they never finished the trial (p. 58).

The trial, as planned, was only five weeks in duration. But according to De Cicco's critical analysis from the in-house FDA meeting, "Fabre has a 4-week trial at the most."

Considering all this, the study should have been discarded as worthless, yet it became one of the cornerstones for approving Prozac.

How did the Prozac patients in the Fabre protocol rate their own response to the drug? They rated themselves no better than the placebo patients rated themselves. In other words, Prozac was no better than placebo from the patients' viewpoint. These negative results occurred despite the placebo washout, which tends to put placebo at a disadvantage compared to the drug. The same critique of the double-blind—that the doctors probably could tell the drug patients from the placebo patients—applies to this and all the FDA Prozac studies.

Meanwhile, is there any reason to question Fabre's integrity? While no legal actions have been brought against him in regard to his studies on Prozac for Eli Lilly, Fabre has recently been accused in a civil suit of gross misconduct in regard to testing Halcion for the Upjohn Company.[9] He is charged, along with Upjohn, with participation in a "conspiracy, first to market Halcion and keep Halcion . . . on the market." In regard to studies he conducted for Upjohn from 1973 to 1975, he is accused of the following:

> All of the studies done by Dr. Fabre at the Portland Clinic were falsified. The studies were not "double blind," as they should have been; the drugs were decoded, and both the patient and the investigator knew what drugs the patients were taking.

The "Petition and Jury Demand" of the suit, dated December 22, 1993, also charges Fabre with running more than one study at a time on individual patients, so that they were taking multiple drugs, making it impossible "to determine which side effects were a result of which drugs." It also accuses him of having patients participate in one study after another without the required waiting period between medications.

Dr. Fabre and Upjohn have denied all allegations.

Protocol 62: "Seriously Flawed"

According to the FDA's October 3, 1988, "Summary Basis of Approval," Protocol 62 was considered to be the weakest of the three positive protocols. It was also the largest, initially involving 900 patients at ten centers,* although a variety of factors pared the numbers down considerably. The study consisted of two distinct parts, one testing the drug on "mildly" depressed patients and the other "moderately" depressed patients. The following analysis is taken from the Food and Drug Administration "Review and Evaluation of Clinical Data: Amendment," dated December 30, 1985.

On various measurements, including the patients' ratings of themselves, the slightly larger group diagnosed as mildly depressed showed no improvement on Prozac—an observation that becomes more interesting in light of currently publicized claims that Prozac is especially helpful to mildly depressed people. The moderately depressed group included only 171 Prozac patients who actually completed the six-week trial. The moderately depressed patients did show some improvement, including on their subjective rating of themselves.[10] There were no seriously depressed patients in the protocol.

In Protocol 62, the dropout rates were high in all dose ranges: over 35 percent at 20 mgs., over 40 percent at 40 mgs., and over 50 percent at 60 mgs. The most common reason for dropping out was adverse side effects and the second was lack of effectiveness. The most frequent side effects were nervousness, anxiety, insomnia, nausea, an-

*The principal investigators were Roland J. Branconnier, Ph.D., and Eric Dessain, M.D.; Jay B. Cohn, M.D., Ph.D.; M. Lynn Crimson, Pharm.D., and Allen Childs, M.D.; David L. Dunner, M.D.; Louis F. Fabre, Jr., M.D., Ph.D.; John P. Feighner, M.D.; Roland R. Fieve, M.D.; Joseph Mendels, M.D.; Ram K. Shrivastava, M.D.; Ward T. Smith, M.D.

orexia, and diarrhea, *each of which occurred in more than 15 percent of patients.* Even at the lowest dose, more than 70 percent of the patients experienced at least one side effect, and at the highest dose, 90 percent endured one or more.

The FDA is very critical of this protocol. It was unable to identify a specific "time period when the results became significant." There were no significant differences between the drug and the placebo before the fourth week. According to the December 30, 1985, FDA evaluation, this study was so "seriously flawed" in design that interpretation was difficult (pp. 12 and 13). The concluding line of the FDA's amended analysis states, "It is not possible to arrive at a single, unequivocal interpretation of the results."[11] Keep in mind that this protocol, like the others, used the placebo-washout strategy that skews the results in favor of the drug, and that this protocol was one of the three most positive in a much larger field of negative protocols.

As already noted in regard to Protocol 27, both Feighner and Cohn were seriously criticized by the FDA on various grounds. Both were principal investigators in Protocol 62. Fabre, whose legal situation we discussed in regard to Protocol 19, was also a principal investigator in Protocol 62.

Fieve Presents a Different View of Protocol 62

One of Lilly's hand-picked principal investigators in the ten-site Protocol 62 was psychiatrist Ronald R. Fieve, a professor at Columbia University and chief of psychiatric research at the New York State Psychiatric Institute. Fieve is the author of the 1994 mass-market book *Prozac: Questions and Answers for Patients, Family, and Physicians.*

In the preface to his book, Fieve describes how eager he was to participate as one of Eli Lilly's principal investigators and he tells the reader that the protocol did obtain the anticipated positive result for Prozac. But his analysis of Protocol 62 bears little resemblance to the facts on several critical points:

Fieve says that the protocol included a comparison antidepressant, Tofranil, but it did not.[12]

Fieve states that the "pooled data" showed that Prozac worked better than placebo. As noted, there were two studies, and the pooled data for the mildly depressed patients showed no efficacy. A positive effect was barely measured only for the moderately depressed patients, a factor Fieve does not share with the reader. And, of course, there were no seriously depressed patients in the study, another fact Fieve does not share with the reader.

Fieve states that "Prozac patients experienced a startling absence of side effects compared to imipramine patients." Not only were there no imipramine patients for comparison, adverse side effects afflicted the vast majority of Prozac patients and helped to cause a very substantial drop-out rate.

Fieve says that Prozac was proven as effective as the older antidepressant, Tofranil, when the latter wasn't even included.

Elsewhere in his book, without citing the FDA studies, Fieve states "approximately 65% to 70% of depressed patients who take their Prozac are fully relieved within two to six weeks. . . ." But he couldn't have concluded this from Protocol 62 or from any other Lilly-sponsored FDA study of Prozac. The high drop-out rates in all those research projects make it impossible to conclude that 65 to 70 percent of the patients were improved. At least one-third of the patients usually failed to finish the trials and drop-out rates sometimes reach 50 percent. Besides, the vast majority of protocols and individual studies showed no positive effect from Prozac.

In a telephone interview on April 6, 1994, I asked Fieve to clarify the discrepancies. Initially, Fieve thought he recalled an antidepressant control group in his Lilly-sponsored FDA study; but after taking a moment to check with his assistant, he acknowledged that his memory had been inaccurate. He thanked me and said that he would fix the error in the next edition of his book.

In the interview, Fieve repeated that other FDA studies did prove Prozac to be as effective as the older antidepressants, and was surprised when I assured him that in fact Prozac consistently proved less effective according to the FDA. Fieve's misperception about this is understandable, since *Lilly's* (as opposed to the FDA's) published version of Protocol 27, as we have already noted, claimed that the drugs did show comparable efficacy. Almost no one reads the FDA's analysis, which must be obtained through the Freedom of Information Act.

When I reminded Fieve, he acknowledged that his Lilly-sponsored Prozac study showed no positive effect on more than half the patients in his study—those diagnosed as mildly depressed—and that the FDA found the whole study very flawed.

I asked Fieve how he could write in his book that up to 70 percent of patients will improve on Prozac when the FDA studies showed that up to 50 percent were likely to drop out due to adverse effects and lack of efficacy. The numbers were contradictory.

Fieve explained that the 70 percent improvement rate cited in his book was based on his personal impressions from his extensive clinical practice in which he gives Prozac and other SSRIs to most of his depressed patients. When pressed, he said that the 70 percent estimate did not include the one-third of his Prozac patients who dropped out, mainly due to adverse side effects. He explained that the 70 percent improvement rate was based on those patients *who remain on the drug,* not on all the patients who start taking the drug. But simple math shows that's an improvement rate of only 47 percent[13]—less than placebo in many studies.*

*But even these relatively unimpressive improvement rates cannot be

Prozac Plus?

In chapter 4, we shall find that stimulant effects—including insomnia, nightmares, agitation, anxiety, and nervousness—are very commonly caused by SSRIs, especially Prozac. To counteract these adverse effects, clinicians frequently prescribe an additional drug along with Prozac. These include sleeping pills, such as chloral hydrate, or benzodiazepines (minor tranquilizers), such as Klonopin, Dalmane, or Xanax. Sometimes the sedative is prescribed with the first dose of the SSRI, sometimes it is prescribed only after stimulant symptoms, such as insomnia or agitation, begin to appear. Either way, the patient is exposed not only to the hazards of SSRIs but to those of sleeping pills and minor tranquilizers, which include addiction, withdrawal, and mental dysfunction.

In setting up and carrying out its protocols, Lilly seemed to recognize that some Prozac patients would also need to be put on sedatives or tranquilizers. According to the FDA's March 28, 1985, report, Protocol 27 states that patients will be excluded from the study if they take psychotropic drugs "other than benzodiazepines or chloral hydrate" (p. 5). Under "concomitant medications," the protocol seems to set a more narrow spectrum of permissible sedatives, stating that the only allowable medications were choral hydrate or flurazepam (Dalmane) for sleep.

In Protocol 19, patients were supposed to be excluded if they took any other psychoactive drugs (p. 52). However, there is a seeming contradiction, because under con-

---

taken too seriously, because clinical impressions from one's own practice are easily distorted to meet personal expectations or hopes. That's why controlled studies are required. It is not sound to publish subjective personal estimates in a book as if they have scientific validity. It is especially inappropriate not to delineate between clinical impression and empirical data when it comes to providing scientific-sounding percentages.

comitant medications, it is stated that "According to the protocol, the only allowable concomitant medication was chloral hydrate for sleep and benzodiazepines (not further specified) for agitation" (p. 54).

In Protocol 62, as described in the FDA's December 30, 1985, report, patients were supposed to be excluded if they took any additional drug except chloral hydrate. However, in "actual practice" patients were not excluded if they took benzodiazepines (p. 2).

It is obviously important to know how many of the patients taking Prozac in the FDA trials were in fact taking Prozac plus a sedative, yet the numbers involved are not reported in Protocols 19, 27, or 62. However, during one of the attempts to pool the data for Protocol 27, Lilly decided to exclude all patients who took other drugs. According to the FDA's March 28, 1985, report, it turned out that patients were taking a wide variety of sedative drugs, including sedative tricyclic antidepressants, phenobarbital, and benzodiazepines (p. 48). Not counting the Cohn study, which had been dropped, 25 percent (135 of 540) of the enrolled patients were taking an additional drug.

Of critical importance is that when patients taking sedative drugs were removed from the pooled data, Prozac failed to show significant efficacy. Prozac proved efficacious only when patients taking the additional sedative drugs were reincluded in the pool (p. 50-A).

The inclusion of sedative drugs in Lilly's approval studies completely distorts them. In effect, the FDA ended up approving Prozac in combination with sedatives.

Prozac's Tests Show it to Be Anything But a Miracle Cure

To sum up, the three protocols we have examined were the only ones that the FDA judged valid enough to use for demonstrating efficacy. A large number of other studies were even more scientifically questionable or showed Prozac to be ineffective. These three badly flawed efforts, with many patients suffering adverse reactions, are the basis for the FDA allowing Prozac to be given to millions of Americans. A lot of fancy numbers-crunching was required to make Prozac look any better than a lowly sugar pill. In addition, several of the investigators were severely criticized by the FDA for their practices, including failure to observe protocol rules.

It bears repeating: These three protocols—with only 286 Prozac patients finishing the four- to six-week studies—were the best that Eli Lilly and the FDA could come up with to prove the value of Prozac.

We believe the FDA, based on its analyses, should not have approved Prozac. All in all, this is anything but an encouraging outcome for the drug—hardly the stuff national crazes are made of. We will have to keep looking for the real underlying causes of Prozac's enthusiastic endorsement by so many patients.

IS THERE ANY SUCH DRUG AS AN ANTIDEPRESSANT?

Recently the whole idea of an antidepressant drug has been challenged. If you believe, as we do, that depression is a form of psychological suffering based on hopelessness and despair, it would seem unlikely that drugging the brain could substantially help. On the other hand, any drug, including a sugar pill, might help by providing hope and encouragement, especially if the doctor offers it with authority and enthusiasm, and even more especially if the media are pushing it as well.

These observations have been recently confirmed in a series of new studies by psychologists Roger Greenberg, Ph.D., and Seymour Fisher, Ph.D. Both Greenberg and Fisher are professors at the Department of Psychiatry and Behavioral Sciences of the State University of New York

Health Sciences Center in Syracuse.[14] In 1992 a team led by Greenberg performed a statistical meta-analysis of 22 independent double-blind studies of three relatively new antidepressant drugs—Asendin (amoxapine), Ludiomil (maprotiline), and Desyrel (trazodone). Each study included both a placebo group and a comparison to an older drug.

According to self-ratings by the patients in these studies, the newer and older antidepressants were no better than placebo. In the words of Greenberg and his research team, "Thus, patient ratings of outcome for both standard and new antidepressant medication showed virtually no benefit beyond that obtained from placebo."*

While clinician ratings of patient improvement were a little more positive, Greenberg's research casts serious doubt on these evaluations. Studies show that clinicians are often able to guess who is receiving the drug and who is getting the sugar pill. Patients can also be influenced by side effects that inform them whether or not they are ingesting an active substance. They naturally feel more improved by an agent that has solid side effects.

To make a fair comparison between a drug and a placebo, the sugar pill needs a little punch of its own, something to make the patient think a real treatment is taking place. When patients are given active or enhanced placebos—drugs, such as atropine, that have side effects but no antidepressant effect—the patients improve as much as if they were on so-called antidepressants. In a 1993 report, Fisher and Greenberg concluded that it's time to view with skepticism any study in which the placebo does not have significant side effects.†

In discussing the study, Greenberg told Bruce Bower of *Science News* that an unpublished meta-analysis by himself and Fisher showed Prozac to be no better than

---

*In contrast, Greenberg finds that studies of psychotherapy for depression demonstrate improvement on both patient and clinician ratings.
†I came to the same conclusion in *Toxic Psychiatry* (1991).

any of the other antidepressant drugs, all of which had doubtful efficacy.

Despite the current enthusiasm for Prozac, the FDA studies underscored the drug's lack of effectiveness, and recent analyses of literature indicate that antidepressants in general are no better than placebo. But placebo, as Fisher and Greenberg reconfirmed, is very powerful. The lowly sugar pill—utterly free of brain-disabling and life-threatening adverse effects—improves a large portion of depressed patients.* It may be the true miracle.

If Prozac isn't very effective, is it at least relatively safe? That was the hope within psychiatry when Prozac gained FDA approval. If it wasn't anything special therapeutically, it might have fewer or less serious side effects than other antidepressants. In the next three chapters, we turn to adverse reactions caused by Prozac, a subject of ultimately greater concern to consumers than Prozac's ineffectiveness as an antidepressant.

*Patients do frequently report side effects when taking placebo, but however real the effects seem, they do not cause actual brain dysfunction and damage or threaten the individual's life.

FOUR

The Real Story Behind Prozac's Side Effects

Tammy calls herself a down-home girl, reared on a farm near a small midwestern town of fewer than 200 souls. She's chunky and brashly dressed in red stretch pants and a colorful patchwork shirt borrowed from her aunt. She's a green-eyed blonde, open, direct, and no-nonsense. At age twenty-two, she's already the mother of three children.

The birth of Tammy's third child, plus a bad virus that she couldn't shake, left her feeling exhausted and overwhelmed. She couldn't get out of bed and didn't want to be bothered with the kids. Disparaging herself in retrospect, she explains, "I was feeling sorry for myself." The family was also going through hard times, she says. "We were dirt poor."

After a few weeks, Tammy's general practitioner decided Prozac might be the best thing for her, and "to give me a jump start," he prescribed two capsules a day. For a few days, she felt great, but within a few more, she began to change. "I couldn't sleep. Monsters came into my head, trying to tell me that I just didn't want to live." Then she explains with genuine humiliation and grief. "I wanted to kill my kids. I decided I couldn't kill myself and leave them behind, so it was easier and better to kill them, too. It makes me feel sick to say it, Dr. Breggin.

My husband had guns. It probably would have been with a gun."

Nighttime became nightmare time for Tammy. "I didn't want to go to bed because every night I wondered if that would be the one when the monsters really took over. During the day, I'd eat to bury everything and during the night it would happen all over again."

Tammy had never been depressed before, never suicidal: "I'm totally against suicide. I don't personally believe in it. If you're going to take your own life, you're thinking of no one but yourself. It's very selfish." It was also the only time she'd had murderous feelings toward her children.

While taking Prozac, Tammy had no idea it was doing anything to her mind. She thought her awful feelings were part of being depressed. And although the contradiction didn't make any sense, at the same time she thought she was doing great—better than ever. She invested $500—a small fortune by her family's standards—in a "get-rich-quick" scheme to sell a diet plan, and ultimately lost all her investment.

"I lost all my friends," she explained. "I didn't want any. Hey, I was indispensable. How can anybody survive without me? Felt like I didn't need anybody. People just pissed me off really easy and I didn't want them around."

Tammy started eating and smoking obsessively. Now, several years later, she has not returned to her normal weight.

Although she never told anyone about her nightmarish feelings, Tammy's mother, father, and husband saw changes in her. "My friends and family knew I was getting weird. They said I was moody, snippy, and real full of myself, arrogant." But she didn't listen. She would clam up, get angry, and storm out.

Because it was too expensive for her, Tammy stopped taking Prozac after three months and gradually over the next few months she began to "snap out of it." Then she started feeling guilty about having wanted to hurt herself and her three children, and she still reproaches herself about it. Otherwise she is back to her "old perky, high-energy me."

Still not realizing she'd undergone a Prozac reaction, a year later Tammy read an article about another woman's experience on the drug, and "it sounded just like me." The woman in the story had been plotting to commit suicide and also had become obsessive and compulsive.

A pattern emerges from one story after another. Often it begins with people feeling better—sometimes better than ever. Then other things begin to happen—violent or suicidal feelings that seem alien but compelling, obsessions and compulsions, impulsive and often grandiose behaviors, and especially a lack of empathy for oneself and others—a human disconnection.

"Have they put a warning on the bottle about it yet?" Tammy asked me, and I had to answer, "No."

"How come?" she asked in dismay.

HOW A DRUG'S LABEL IS CREATED

Most people tend to "believe in" or trust the list of drug side effects found in a medical source book or in the package insert that comes along with the bottle. The average person has little idea that the creation of that list of adverse drug reactions has much to do with the politics of what I call the psycho-pharmaceutical complex, and often very little to do with the health and safety of the consumer.

The FDA's powers derive from its mandate to supervise the labeling of drugs. In order to be marketed in the United States, a new drug must have an FDA-approved label concerning safety and efficacy. The label must appear in its entirety in the *Physicians' Desk Reference* and in the insert that goes along with bottles of the medication. In a modified form that emphasizes adverse effects and other dangers, it must appear as well with all forms of advertising, typically on the back side of the gaudy ads that appear in journals and consumer publications.

As we discussed in chapter 3, to obtain an approved label, the drug company—called the sponsor—must undertake and report a series of studies, culminating in scientifically controlled comparisons of the new drug to established drugs and to placebo, or "sugar pill." The scientifically controlled studies, called Phase III, are usually only four to six weeks in duration.

The drug company also presents anecdotal data from lengthier, uncontrolled studies, as well as from individual clinical reports. These less scientifically refined data continue to flow in after the drug has been marketed.

As already described in chapter 3, the FDA has no money to finance research carried on during any part of the approval process. The projects are formulated by the manufacturer (Eli Lilly in the case of Prozac) and carried out by doctors of their own choosing, usually physicians with whom the drug company has long-standing professional and financial relationships, and friendly rapport. For the most part, the premarketing studies used for evaluating adverse drug effects are the same ones used for demonstrating efficacy.

Naturally, any profit-making corporation is likely to do everything it can to maximize the possibility that its tests will turn out positive for their drug. After all, millions and perhaps billions of dollars are at stake. Any company would, of course, select physicians and researchers who seem likely to look favorably upon the company's interests. The company will construct the studies so that they are likely to make the drug look good. That's probably why Lilly carried out very few studies on hospitalized patients and excluded any patients with marked suicidal tendencies. The company knew that once the drug came out, physicians would act as if it were a proven treatment for the most difficult patients.

THE REAL FREQUENCY OF ADVERSE REACTIONS IS MUCH HIGHER THAN INDICATED

As we survey the reported rates of side effects, largely derived from Lilly's premarketing studies for the FDA, keep in mind that most of these patients were treated with the relatively low starting dose of 20 mgs. per day and for a very short period of time, rarely exceeding six weeks. Undoubtedly, the rate and severity of side effects—from rashes to mania—would be much greater if the patients were subjected to more typical treatment conditions, including much lengthier periods of exposure to the drugs, the taking of multiple drugs at the same time, and less frequent contacts with the doctor. The patients in the study also were physically healthy, whereas, in the real world, patients often receive antidepressants while suffering from and being treated for many different physical disorders.

A side effect is likely to be noticed relatively quickly in a drug study, compared to routine clinical practice, and drug treatment will be stopped before really serious problems develop. But when a patient doesn't see the doctor for weeks or months at a time, as too frequently happens in the real world, seemingly minor side effects can mushroom into serious problems.

During drug-testing trials, it is relatively uncommon to use combinations of several drugs, yet this is commonplace in clinical practice. When drugs have been prescribed along with Prozac, or along with any psychoactive medication, the odds of unexpected complications or side effects vastly increase. Again, the premarket testing procedures cannot adequately detect dangers that will be associated with the routine clinical use of the drug, and, as we shall see, this has already proven so with Prozac.

The relatively short duration of the controlled studies—

four to six weeks—almost guarantees that even very serious adverse effects will be undetected before marketing if they take months or years to develop. Consider the negative effects of smoking tobacco or drinking alcohol. If these drugs were tested like Prozac in moderate doses for only a few weeks on a few thousand people, almost none of the more serious side effects would show up. Lung cancer, emphysema, gastrointestinal disorders, and circulatory diseases, to name but a few of tobacco's adverse effects, typically don't show until after years of smoking. While the intoxicating effects of relatively large doses of alcohol are quickly apparent, brain and liver disease, among other disorders, may not show up for decades.

According to Lilly's account in the *Physicians' Desk Reference,* the pooled data for adverse reactions from all the premarketing studies in the case of Prozac involved approximately 4,000 patients. But this is not a sufficiently large number to screen for relatively uncommon dangerous drug reactions. A fatal reaction that occurs on the average only once in every 4,000 Prozac patients, for example, might not turn up at all. If it did occur once or twice, it could easily be dismissed as being unrelated to the drug. Yet that adverse reaction could end up causing the deaths of 1,000 among the first 4 million patients treated with the drug.

Equally important, pooled data does not adequately detect adverse reactions. If, for example, a dozen fatal drug reactions are sprinkled among the 4,000 drug-treated patients in the clinical trials, these disasters might be missed as well. Only a few of the individual research studies would encounter even one of these deaths. Those studies that did experience a fatality would be unaware of the overall pattern and might easily fail to attribute the single case to a drug reaction. This may have contributed to what happened in a controversial, ill-fated Lilly study of an anti-hepatitis pill where, in the early stages of testing, several drug-related deaths were mistakenly attributed to other causes and not even reported to the FDA.[1]

Perhaps most important, if the disastrous effect takes a few months or years to develop, it will not show up in the four- to six-week studies, and is likely to be overlooked during the testing. And in the case of Prozac, on top of that, a large percentage of the 4,000 patients who received the drug in the clinical trials dropped out early in the research studies.

As a result of the limitations built into the premarketing studies, many serious adverse drug reactions do not show up until after a drug has been marketed. In April 1990, the United States General Accounting Office (GAO), a congressional watchdog agency, reviewed all drugs approved by the FDA between 1976 and 1985. It found that 102 of 198 approved drugs turned out to have "serious postapproval risks"—"adverse reactions that could lead to hospitalization, increases in the length of hospitalization, severe or permanent disability, or death."

The rate was even higher for psychiatric drugs: Nine of fifteen recently approved medications developed serious postapproval risks, including one that had to be withdrawn from the market. Four relatively new antidepressants—Asendin (amoxapine), Wellbutrin (buproprion), Ludiomil (maprotiline), and Desyrel (trazodone)—were among those requiring major label changes. A fifth antidepressant, Merital (nomifensine), was withdrawn from the market after it was found to cause potentially fatal immune-system disorders. The minor tranquilizer Xanax (alprazolam), sometimes used as an antidepressant, had paradoxical rage reactions added to its label. For reasons that are not clear, antidepressants seem to have the highest probability of slipping through the FDA screening process with undetected serious and even life-threatening adverse effects.

In all categories, the GAO found that six drugs were no longer approved and the remainder had changes in labeling. The GAO also noted that it can take several years for the FDA to act upon risks that are identified in the postapproval period.

When we examine the evaluation of Prozac-related violence and suicide, we will take a much closer look at the entire process whereby adverse reaction reports are gathered once drug marketing has begun.

WHAT PROZAC'S LABEL WON'T TELL YOU

The FDA's supervisory function over the pharmaceutical industry is exercised largely through its control over the label that becomes attached to an approved drug. According to FDA regulations, the label must contain the following sections: description, clinical pharmacology, indications and usage, contraindications, warnings, precautions, adverse reactions, drug abuse and dependence, overdosage, dosage and administration, and how supplied. Each of those categories has potential relevance to hazards and adverse drug reactions. As the data is collected during the premarketing evaluation of a drug, the FDA works out a label with representatives of the drug company. It is a give-and-take process.*

Prozac Acts Like A Stimulant

After all the data had been collected during Prozac's approval process, FDA psychiatrist Richard Kapit wrote the official "Safety Review" of adverse reactions or side effects. Drawing on the Lilly-sponsored studies and more general sources of information, Kapit made the definitive evaluation of the type, frequency, and severity of negative drug effects. Kapit's bosses at the FDA, especially psychiatrist Paul Leber, head of the department that evaluates psycho-pharmaceuticals, would have the final say, but Kapit was the expert analyst who put it all together and made the formal analysis. Fortunately, Kapit's report was

*For the politics of that process, see chapter 7.

made available to us through the Freedom of Information Act.

In the abstract on the first page of his final report, Kapit stated "most frequently this new drug caused nausea, insomnia, and nervousness, which resembles the profile of a stimulant rather than a sedative drug." He thought this stimulant profile would "give rise to the greatest clinical liabilities in the use of this medication," including "insomnia, nervousness, anorexia, and weight loss."

There is additional support in Kapit's report for viewing Prozac as a stimulant. The Lilly data confirms additional stimulant-type side effects: "agitation, irritability, excitement," nightmares, sweating, dry mouth, abnormal sensations, abnormal bodily movements, and palpitations. In addition, a small percentage of patients suffered psychotic reactions, usually hypomania or mania, a reaction consistent with central nervous system overstimulation.* And finally, overdoses of Prozac were found to produce brain stimulation, including seizures, "hypomania, agitation, restlessness, and other signs of CNS [central nervous system] excitation."[2] Later in his report, Kapit repeated his observations, stating that Prozac's "profile of adverse effects more closely resembles that of a stimulant drug than one that causes sedation and gain of weight."

The FDA psychiatrist was also concerned that some of Prozac's stimulant properties might contribute to a worsening of depression. He warned that, "Since depressed patients frequently suffer from insomnia, nervousness, anorexia, and weight loss, it is possible that fluoxetine treatment might, at least temporarily, make their illness

---

*Mania and its more mild form, hypomania, are serious mental disturbances in which the individual becomes euphoric, hyperactive, and driven by grandiose or unrealistic appraisals of his or her own power and abilities. Judgment and insight are impaired, and impulsivity dominates. Typically there is a "flight of ideas" as the mind races out of control. Often there is paranoia, hostility, and sometimes violence. Insomnia and exhaustion are common, and the individual may lapse into depression.

worse." At the conclusion of his review, Kapit repeated the warning that Prozac might, in some cases, worsen depression.

What did the FDA do regarding their reviewer's warnings about the dangers of the stimulant profile and the associated risk of worsening depression? They expunged Kapit's conclusions from the drug's label. Nowhere in the basic information that must appear in the *Physicians' Desk Reference* and in all advertising is Eli Lilly required to indicate that Prozac is a stimulant drug or that it can cause or worsen depression.

Why did the FDA decide to edit out the most significant and often-repeated observations and warnings of its own official reviewer? When I interviewed Kapit in 1991, he could not or would not tell me. But as we proceed through this book, the reader will hear more evidence about how avidly the FDA supports the drug industry and its needs at the expense of the public and the consumer.

After the FDA approved Prozac in December 1987, it continued to negotiate with Eli Lilly concerning its label, and on March 4, 1988, Kapit wrote a memorandum concerning proposed last-minute revisions for the Prozac label.[3] It drew upon Lilly's data base for the 5,620 U.S. patients treated with Prozac as of July 31, 1987.* Kapit stated that Lilly's estimates of frequencies for side effects in general were unsuitable for inclusion in the revision "since the method used by the company to derive these numbers was inappropriate," but his memo doesn't describe the specific problems with Lilly's approach.

Kapit also continued to call for some attention to stimulant effects in the official label. For example, he requested that Lilly include a table that would organize

---

* This is probably the same figure described in the drug label as 5,600 "Prozac-exposed" individuals in the premarketing period (see chapter 3).

stimulant symptoms in a comprehensible fashion. His efforts were to no avail, apparently overridden by his superiors.

In "Conclusions and Recommendations," Kapit warned:

> To this reviewer's eyes, the tables proposed by Lilly will be too large and will contain too much extraneous information and noise. Many of the ADR [adverse drug reaction] columns are not relevant. It is almost a fact of physics that the more noise in a signal, the more difficult it will be to extract information from it.*

The noise in the chart, as Kapit worried, is enormously distracting. Why, for example, list symptoms unrelated to the drug effect, such as "nasal congestion," which appeared almost equally in the Prozac and control patients? Why list "cough" or "chest pain" when it's no more frequent than in placebo? As Kapit said, if you put enough extraneous material in a chart, people cannot grasp the significance of what is there. In this case, the significance includes Prozac's stimulant profile.

Kapit's memo discussed the possibility of introducing two specialized tables, one of which would summarize the stimulant effects of Prozac. Kapit concluded by stating that he would discuss his recommendations with his boss, Paul Leber.

What can we presume was the outcome of his discussions with Leber, whose name will appear again when we examine the highly biased FDA hearings on violence and suicide from Prozac? Kapit's suggestions never came to fruition and the Prozac label, as found in the package

---

*Kapit also felt that if the largest tables were "sanctioned" by the FDA, "then the company [Eli Lilly] will be free to perform whatever analysis of the table they wish; the larger the table, and the greater the amount of extraneous information, the more likely it becomes that spurious results will be generated."

insert and the *Physicians' Desk Reference,* contains a huge table with dozens of side effects organized by systems of the body, providing no hint of a coherent pattern of stimulant effects.

CONFIRMING THE STIMULANT SYNDROME FROM THE PDR TABLE OF ADVERSE DRUG EFFECTS

The *PDR* table* of Prozac's side effects organizes them according to systems of the body, starting in order with the nervous system, the digestive system, and the skin. *Nearly all* of the symptoms reported in these three organ systems fit into the stimulant syndrome.

The following "Nervous System Symptoms" associated with Prozac, listed in the table, are indistinguishable from those associated with amphetamine or cocaine:[4]

    headache (20.3 percent)
    nervousness (14.9 percent)
    insomnia (13.8 percent)
    anxiety (9.4 percent)
    tremor (7.9 percent)

As less-frequent nervous system side effects, the table also lists dizziness, light-headedness, and decreased concentration, all of which can also be caused by stimulant drugs. Under nervous system effects, the table also lists drowsiness (11.6 percent), fatigue (4.2 percent), and sedation (1.9 percent). While these are the opposite of a stimulant syndrome, they also occur in patients taking drugs such as amphetamines and cocaine. They result from the brain's attempt to react against the stimulation.

The *PDR* list of drug-induced digestive symptoms is im-

---

*The table is based on "placebo-controlled clinical trials" with 1,730 patients who received Prozac (see chapter 3).

posing* and is also wholly consistent with stimulant drugs, such as amphetamines and cocaine:

nausea (21.1 percent)
diarrhea (12.3 percent)
mouth dryness (9.5 percent)
anorexia (8.7 percent)
dyspepsia (6.4 percent)
abdominal pain (3.4 percent)
vomiting (2.4 percent)

Under "Skin and Appendages," the table also lists "excessive sweating (8.4 percent)," another common finding with stimulant drugs.

If we examine every symptom in the table that appears substantially more often with Prozac than with placebo, every one of them is a stimulant-profile side effect.† But the physician scanning the table is not likely to draw this information from it.

The most direct suggestion of a stimulant syndrome is found in the text of the label under the "Precautions" section. "Anxiety, nervousness, and insomnia"— all stimulant reactions—are reported as occurring in 10 to 15 percent of patients, leading 5 percent to discontinue the drug.

Important information that might have underscored the stimulant syndrome does not appear in the *PDR* table but is buried elsewhere in the label. For example, agitation and nightmares are missing from the table, yet in the "Adverse Reactions" section of the label, under "Nerv-

---

*The table distracts from the total percentage of patients suffering gastrointestinal complaint by listing eleven separate categories of effects. Glancing at it, the physician is not likely to realize that the proportion of patients with a variation of stomach discomfort *exceeds 50 percent*. Some of these reports may overlap, but most likely most of them represent individual patients.

†My criterion was a rate approximately 4 percent higher for Prozac than placebo.

ous System," abnormal dreams and agitation are listed as frequent.*

Also missing from the table, but found in the "Precautions" section, is the observation that mania and hypomania, typical stimulant reactions, occurred in approximately 1 percent of patients.

Similarly, the classic stimulant side effect of weight loss is absent from the table; but under "Precautions," the label states, "Significant weight loss, especially in underweight depressed patients, may be an undesirable result of treatment with Prozac." Thirteen percent of Prozac-treated patients lost weight in excess of 5 percent of their body weight.

A list of all the stimulant symptoms mentioned in various parts of the label should have been put into one table. It would have looked like this:

THE PROZAC STIMULANT PROFILE

I. Psychiatric and Neurological
headache (20.3 percent)
nervousness (14.9 percent)
insomnia (13.8 percent)
anxiety (9.4 percent)
tremor (7.9 percent)
hypomania and mania (1 percent)
agitation (frequent)
abnormal dreams (frequent)
seizures (0.2 percent)

II. Digestive System
significant weight loss (13 percent)
nausea (21.1 percent)
diarrhea (12.3 percent)
mouth dryness (9.5 percent)
anorexia (8.7 percent)
dyspepsia (6.4 percent)

*Frequent in the FDA literature means "occurring in at least one in one hundred" patients treated with the drug in question.

abdominal pain (3.4 percent)
vomiting (2.4 percent)

III. Skin
excessive sweating (8.4 percent)

As we shall document, the stimulant profile should also have included another category:

IV. Behavioral
paranoia
violence
depression ("crashing")
suicide
drug abuse

It is relatively easy to remember most of the main side effects of SSRIs—Prozac, Zoloft, and Paxil—simply by keeping in mind the principle of stimulation or activation. Only time will tell whether Zoloft and Paxil vary significantly from Prozac in their profile of stimulant effects. Since these drugs are even more potent blockers of serotonin reuptake, it seems unlikely that their adverse effects will be more benign.

THE LILLY TRIALS MASK THE RATES OF STIMULANT SIDE EFFECTS

Although Kapit does not mention it, there is strong evidence that the rates of stimulant side effects, such as anxiety, nervousness, and insomnia, were much higher than those reported by the Lilly investigators. According to the FDA in-house reports, patients in Protocol 27 and Protocol 19 could be treated with minor tranquilizers, such as Valium, Ativan, and Xanax, as well as with the sedative chloral hydrate, during the Prozac trials. Patients in Protocol 62 were only supposed to receive chloral hydrate but in practice were not excluded if they received minor tranquilizers (see chapter 3).

These additional drugs were given to a significant but only partially documented number of patients. Data associated with the first attempt to pool the results of Protocol 27 shows that additional drugs were given to 142 of the 706 patients initially enrolled in the studies. While some of the patients "erroneously" received unapproved medications, these unapproved drugs turn out to be antidepressants with sedative qualities. As already noted, in Protocol 19 an unspecified number of patients were given minor tranquilizers for agitation.

These tranquilizing and sedative medications would have masked or suppressed the stimulant symptoms caused by Prozac. Since these were the only additional drugs specifically allowed for patients in the Prozac trials, it would seem that Eli Lilly anticipated the need to control the stimulant side effects of Prozac.

The stimulation effects of Prozac, meanwhile, are becoming a well-known problem for clinicians. Research psychiatrist Robert DuPont of the Institute for Behavior and Health, Inc., Rockville, Maryland, has recently sent out a "Dear Doctor" letter seeking patients who have experienced "activation side effects" from Prozac, including "restlessness, anxiety, tremor or insomnia." Like most psychopharmacology advocates who emphasize a drug's negative profile, DuPont is contrasting it to a new and hopefully less troublesome agent that he's testing in clinical trials.

It remains enormously important for the medical profession and the public to learn about Prozac's stimulant profile. This knowledge could still help to protect patients from stimulant-syndrome disasters on Prozac, including paranoia and violence, and crashing with depression and suicide, as well as drug abuse.

Suzanne Robbins, for example, told the following story at the 1991 FDA hearing on Prozac:

I am the head of the Indiana Prozac Survivors Group. . . . I was prescribed Prozac following surgery that had upset my exercise routine and left me feeling just like the doctor said, "a little blue." I had never taken an antidepressant before, so I asked about the possible side effects. He told me the drug was so safe it should be put into the drinking water.

My first reaction came at two weeks. I remember sitting in the car and I reached over and grabbed my husband and said, "I feel like I'm dying." I felt like I was leaving my body. The feeling passed in about 30 seconds, so I thought no more about it.

I was sitting in a classroom two days later when all of a sudden it happened again, only this time I'm shaking, I'm covered in hives, and my mind is racing faster and faster. You can't grab the thoughts, they won't stop. I go to the office. I call the doctor. The nurse says, "Oh, let me look in the *PDR*." She looked and said, "Oh, honey, that's not Prozac." I said, "Well, what's happening to me?"

Two more days passed. I was sitting in the classroom again. This time I excused myself from the children. . . . They had to send me home.

I get home and I call the doctor's office again. I said, "I have to see him, something's wrong with me." They said he couldn't see me until Saturday. I said, "You don't understand. Something's wrong with me." He finally saw me the next day, took one look at me, now covered with hives, I'm shaking, I can't think, I can't formulate a thought, and he said, "Oh, you're having a panic attack. It's not Prozac."

So I went home and I thought I'm going to die. There's something really wrong with me. Saturday I went through the day. It was a blur. I just remember feeling strange. On Sunday, I'm a Sunday school teacher. I went to Sunday school and I handed them my Sunday school papers and I said, "Something's wrong with me, I have to get out of here."

I left the church and got into my car and I'm driving the interstate, trying to hold on to the wheel. The thoughts are racing so fast and it's saying "you're going to die," and I have to hold on to the wheel to keep from going off the road. . . .

I finally admitted myself to a stress center. I begged them, "Lock me up because I'm going to die and I don't want to die." The internist walked in, and I remember the day so well, she took one look at me and she said, "Prozac. You're not my first victim." She said, "The last one I saw they had doubled the dose and she was in full psychosis."

I knew at that moment I would live, but I didn't understand the horrors that this drug would not leave my system right away. They had to sit by my bed and they would hold me down as I shook and they would tell me, they would say, "You're going through drug withdrawal." My God, it was horrible. . . .

When Ginger Breggin asked Suzanne if she was depressed at the time of starting Prozac, Suzanne said with emphasis, "No, I was given the drug following foot surgery. I had felt a little down after the surgery because I couldn't exercise and asked the doctor for a pick-me-up."

Ginger Breggin's initial interview with Suzanne disclosed something Suzanne herself had not realized—that her reaction was a classic example of drug-induced central nervous system stimulation. I confirmed this during my follow-up interview.

Although Suzanne had not appreciated the significance of it at the time, and therefore not described it fully in her FDA testimony, her pre-drug fatigue and blues were transformed within days to a constellation of stimulant symptoms, including sleeplessness, nervousness, tremor, inability to sit still, feeling like she couldn't breathe, anxiety, lack of concentration, and a sense of "being dead inside." Despite the deadness inside, she was speeding mentally on Prozac, "like a tape recorder going fast-forward in my head." She lost her appetite and five pounds in the three weeks that she was on the drug. She felt compulsively driven "to do something," but she didn't know what it might be. She said to family or friends, "I have to go, I have to go," but she didn't know where.

Back in the 1960s, Suzanne took diet pill amphetamines

and experienced temporary stimulation effects. She told me, "Everybody took them then. We didn't know the ramifications." She explained, "I remember the diet pill stimulation only lasted about thirty minutes to an hour— that feeling of being driven, of having to do things, and being euphoric. It was a short time. But on Prozac there was constant stimulation. It didn't go away while you were on the drug."* Prozac produced "no instant surge of euphoria" but the underlying "hyper" feeling was similar to the amphetamines.

The two other approved SSRIs—Zoloft and Paxil— tend to produce similar side effects to Prozac, but probably with less intense stimulation, and perhaps more frequent sedation. Like Prozac, neither of their FDA-approved labels contains a specific mention of stimulant effects.

In animal experiments, Paxil is the most potent reuptake blocker of all,[5] suggesting to me that its tendency to cause agitation and other stimulant symptoms may thus far have been underestimated. It is reported to cause a feeling of being "wiped out."

OTHER ADVERSE DRUG REACTIONS

The Prozac label lists a variety of other drug side effects that lie outside the stimulant profile, but that are important hazards. Some of these are adequately described in the label and some are not.

Sexual Dysfunction

In the table in the Lilly label for Prozac, there is a misleading breakdown in categories in regard to sexual prob-

---

*Amphetamines have a much shorter span of activity in the body, accounting for these differences (see chapter 5).

lems. In the left-hand column, under nervous system, decreased libido (1.6 percent) is listed. But in the right-hand column, under urogenital, sexual dysfunction (1.9 percent) appears. It was only after studying the chart for several minutes that I realized Lilly had split sexual disorders into two different columns. But even the combined totals of sexual dysfunction reported in the table has turned out to be drastically underestimated.

After Prozac came out, reports began to estimate the rate of drug-induced sexual dysfunction as high as 16 percent. Then William Patterson, M.D., from Birmingham, Alabama, specifically queried 60 consecutive men being treated in his practice with 20 mgs. Prozac per day. Over a six-month period, he found that an astonishing 75 percent of his male patients reported retarded ejaculation or ejaculatory incompetence. Lowering the dose was helpful and the problem disappeared when the drug was stopped.

In December 1993, a team led by psychiatrist Parks W. Walker from the University of Tennessee concluded, "While the manufacturer's information indicates that sexual dysfunction associated with the serotonin-selective reuptake inhibitor fluoxetine occurs in less than 2%* of patients, recent reports suggest the incidence may be much higher (7.8%–75% incidence of male sexual dysfunction)." The surfacing of data that differs so drastically from Lilly's FDA studies once again underscores their limitations.

One case of prolonged, painful penile erection has been described with Prozac, and the authors of the report, Michael Murray, M.D., and Daniel Hooberman, M.D., from Boston, hypothesize that serotonin may be involved with inducing erections.

There are anecdotal reports about men who placed

---

*The comment, "less than 2% of patients" with sexual dysfunction, confirms that the noise in the Lilly *Physicians' Desk Reference* table makes it difficult to realize that two kinds of sexual dysfunction are listed, adding up to 3.5 percent.

great importance on their sexual satisfaction but who nonetheless seemed relatively unconcerned when unable to function on Prozac. This again suggests the drug's ability to induce emotional indifference and even withdrawal from previously significant relationships and activities. Many people lose their overall interest in their partners while taking these drugs, and while reducing sexual activity, this would not lead them to report dysfunction or abnormalities to the doctors during the clinical trials.

While the rates for female sexual dysfunction induced by SSRIs seem much lower, significant case reports have been appearing, including difficulty reaching orgasm.

Both Paxil and Zoloft have high rates of sexual dysfunction—mostly ejaculatory problems—in men. In the clinical trials of Paxil, 12.9 percent of men had ejaculatory disturbances, mostly delay, and 10 percent had other sexual dysfunctions, including impotence and the inability to achieve orgasm. Among women, 1.8 percent had difficulty reaching orgasm. In the Zoloft trials, 15.5 percent of men were reported to have sexual difficulties, mostly ejaculatory delay, while 1.7 percent of women experienced problems.

Skin Rashes and Immunological Conditions

Under the "Warnings" heading, Prozac's label lists "Rash and Possibly Allergic Events" as the primary item. The rate of 2.7 percent is based on the relatively short-term approval studies. As Kapit summarized in his FDA report, the rashes included uticaria (hives), as well as maculopapular (small, discolored elevations of skin), purpuric (hermorrhagic), and pustular (pimple-like with pus) lesions.

In less than 10 percent of the rashes, according to a March 4, 1988, memo by Kapit, there were signs of more overall bodily illness, including an elevated white count, abnormal liver-function tests, joint pain, edema or swelling in various parts of the body, and fever. (Sometimes these symptoms have also appeared without rash.) There were also cases of rash with associated signs of kidney dysfunction. In a very small number of rashes, there were signs of a severe and potentially life-threatening immunological disorder, sometimes identified as serum sickness or lupus erythematosis. According to the 1994 *PDR,* deaths occurred in association with similar illnesses after marketing of the drug began.

There are a few reports of inflammatory problems involving the blood vessels of various organs (vasculitis). There have been cases of severe allergic reactions with bronchial spasms that compromise respiration (anaphylactoid shock). These events are reported to be very rare.

Bleeding Problems

Prozac disrupts the uptake of serotonin in blood platelets that are critical to the control of bleeding. There are cases of difficulty with blood clotting, leading to tiny hemorrhages (petechiae) into the skin and vaginal bleeding.[6]

Loss of Sodium

Perhaps through interference with the hormone that controls water retention, Prozac has been associated with a drop in the concentration of serum sodium (hyponatremia). Although relatively rare, this can be a serious problem, especially for older patients and those taking medications that also affect sodium retention, such as antidiuretics for hypertension.

Seizures

Seizures occur with all antidepressants, and Lilly's FDA studies reported a relatively low rate of 0.2 percent. But remember that the studies are very short in duration. Patients who already have a seizure problem should try to avoid all antidepressants.

The Zimelidine Syndrome

The zimelidine syndrome was named after an earlier SSRI that proved too dangerous for use in Europe because of its tendency to cause a cluster of serious flu-like symptoms, including headache, fever, chills, and muscle and joint pain. It could also manifest itself with a paralyzing neurological disorder. While rare, there was concern about its development during treatment with Prozac. No cases of the severe neurological disorder showed up during the FDA-testing period for Prozac, but it remains a concern.

IS THERE A CANCER RISK WITH PROZAC?

Some malignant tumors produce serotonin, and Prozac's impact on them, while unproven, has raised concerns that the drug might stimulate their growth. Antidepressants, including Prozac, have recently been found to promote tumor growth in general in animal laboratory research when used in "clinically relevant doses."[7] As reported in the September 1992 *Psychiatric Times,* the FDA is considering the problem. The problem is especially serious because cancer patients do become depressed and nowadays are likely to be prescribed antidepressants.

Members of the Prozac Survivors Support Group believe there are cases of cancer caused by Prozac, but I have not seen any documented cases. The problem is that usually the only way to make the connection is through the sheer number of cases that develop over time.

DRUG INTERACTION

Any psychiatric drug is likely to interact with other non-prescription and prescription drugs in a variety of potentially harmful ways. Many of these adverse interactions will become apparent only after years of experience in clinical practice, and some may go unnoticed indefinitely, because of the tendency to attribute problems to the patient's "mental illness" or factors other than drug interaction.

Prozac and Alcohol

Many clinicians and Prozac survivors have reported behavioral problems when Prozac is combined with alcohol, but there is no mention of this in the Lilly label. Prozac Survivors Support Group members have told us that many patients, while taking Prozac, increase their alcohol intake or return to previous alcohol abuse. Ann Tracy of the Utah group has pointed out that strains of rats bred for a genetic tendency toward alcohol preference have higher serotonin concentrations in their brains, and these levels increase when they drink alcohol regularly.[8] Another study has shown that depletion of serotonin in the brain tends to reduce alcohol intake in rats.[9] This research is suggestive, but not definitive, of a possible correlation between Prozac, enhanced serotonergic activity, and increased desire for alcohol.

While interviewing teenagers who are former drug abusers, we have been told that Prozac can produce a rapid alcohol high if taken simultaneously with as little as one beer, and that "coming down" afterward is more abrupt and severe. Apparently this is widely known and frequently tried among teenagers who experiment with drugs. Anyone using Prozac should be on the alert for the possible development, worsening, or return of alcohol abuse.

Prozac, Monoamine Oxidase Inhibitors (MAOI), and Tryptophan

When combined with other drugs that stimulate the serotonergic system, such as the monoamine oxidase inhibitor (MAOI) antidepressants or tryptophan,* Prozac can produce a well-documented, severe condition called the serotonin syndrome.[10] This disorder looks somewhat like the serotonin stimulant syndrome and shares with it the symptoms of irrational euphoria (hypomania), agitation, confusion, and gastrointestinal upset, including diarrhea. The serotonin syndrome additionally involves overstimulation of the brain stem and spinal cord, producing symptoms not typically seen with the stimulant syndrome, such as fever and chills, severe incoordination, muscle spasms, and hyperactive reflexes.

Because it involves lower centers in the central nervous system, the serotonin syndrome is more physically disabling than the serotonin stimulant syndrome, and renders the individual unable to carry out purposeful activities such as suicide or murder. By contrast, the stimulant syndrome seems more exclusively to involve the higher centers of the brain and it is frequently caused by Prozac alone.

Because Prozac and its active metabolites last a long time in the system, with a half-life of up to nine days for

*The brain synthesizes serotonin from tryptophan, an essential amino acid found in a variety of foods. The ingestion of large amounts of tryptophan increases the production of serotonin.

one of its metabolites, MAOIs should not be administered to patients until at least five weeks or more after discontinuation of Prozac. If a patient has first been on an MAOI, it should be discontinued for at least fourteen days before beginning Prozac.

Prozac and Tricyclic Antidepressants

Psychiatrists and other physicians too frequently combine Prozac with other antidepressants, including the tricyclics such as Tofranil (imipramine) and Elavil (amitriptyline). The combination is extremely dangerous. In a 1992 study conducted in Lilly's own research laboratory by a team led by Richard Bergstrom, Prozac was found to increase the blood concentrations of tricyclics by as much as *ten times*.[11]

The tricyclics become toxic at blood levels not much higher than their therapeutic ones. A tenfold or more increase in concentration of a tricyclic could produce, among other things, a fatal heart arrhythmia, a severe drop in blood pressure, central nervous system depression, or a grand mal seizure. It could also cause abnormal mental reactions, such as confusion, panic, mania, or even depression.

Does Lilly's writeup in the 1994 *PDR* reflect the data generated several years earlier in their own lab? Under Prozac interactions with "other antidepressants," it states, "There have been greater than 2-fold increases" in blood concentrations with the combination of Prozac. The tricyclic antidepressants are not mentioned by name, and the difference between *greater than twofold* and *tenfold or greater* is enormous. It is a potentially lethal difference.[12]

There is yet another complication to combining fluoxetine with tricyclic antidepressants. One sophisticated study of effects on the rat brain shows that the two given together accelerate their joint impact on the neurotransmitter system.[13]

Prozac and Other Drugs

The discussion of drug interactions in the *Physicians' Desk Reference* is extensive and most physicians, let alone the lay reader, will be pressed to understand or remember them. Any time another medication is taken along with Prozac, caution should be exercised, and a careful review should be made of Prozac's drug interaction profile. In addition to those already discussed in this chapter, the following includes some of the more common problems:

Because Prozac and other SSRIs can cause drowsiness, as well as various cognitive impairments in judgment, thinking, and motor skills, patients are warned of potential difficulties if the drugs are taken while carrying out potentially hazardous activities, such as working with machinery or driving a car. The hazards are increased when Prozac, Zoloft, or Paxil are combined with any other drugs that affect mental processes, including sedatives such as alcohol, sleeping pills, and the minor tranquilizers.

By interfering with liver metabolism, Prozac can increase the blood concentration and hence the toxicity of lithium, as well as minor tranquilizers, such as Valium and Xanax.

Taking Prozac with neuroleptic drugs, such as Thorazine, Haldol, and Navane, can cause increased neuroleptic effects, such as apathy and acute neurological side effects. As we shall further describe in regard to neurological side effects, Prozac inhibits dopamine, the main neurotransmitter system suppressed by the neuroleptics.

Prozac can elevate the blood concentrations of anticoagulants and heart medications, including digitalis and digitoxin, increasing their adverse effects, including heart attack.

Insulin adjustments may be required in diabetics who

take Prozac because the antidepressant lowers the blood sugar (hypoglycemia) and on withdrawal can elevate it (hyperglycemia). Low blood sugar can cause anxiety and other emotional reactions.

Electroshock Treatment

Prozac can increase the dangers of electroshock treatment by prolonging the seizure. It should be stopped several weeks before treatment begins.

PROZAC IN PREGNANT AND NURSING MOTHERS

Prozac is excreted into breast milk, but the potential complications have not been evaluated. Studies on pregnant women have not been done. The drug should be avoided by pregnant and nursing mothers.

AKATHISIA, DYSTONIA, AND THE RISK OF PERMANENT NEUROLOGICAL DISORDERS FROM PROZAC

As early as 1979, H. Y. Meltzer and a team at the University of Chicago recognized that Prozac suppresses dopaminergic neurotransmission. Concerned about reports of neurological side effects that seemed to stem from this dopamine suppression, Ross Baldessarini and Elda Marsh from McLean Hospital and Harvard demonstrated the effect in Prozac-treated animal brains in 1990.

Drug-induced disruption of dopamine neurotransmission is known to produce a variety of neurological side effects. The neuroleptic or antipsychotic drugs—such as Haldol, Navane, Thorazine, Mellaril, and Prolixin—are officially approved for the treatment of severely disturbed psychiatric patients, especially those labeled schizophrenic and acutely manic.* They are, however, frequently used for the outright subjugation of difficult inmates or residents of children's facilities, institutions for the developmentally disabled, nursing homes, board and care homes, and prisons.

The neuroleptics suppress dopamine neurotransmission, initially causing a reversible parkinsonism syndrome with a tremor, shuffling gait, slowed movements, flat facial expression, and dulled or apathetic emotions. A variety of other neuroleptic-induced neurological disorders cause loss of control of the voluntary muscles, including spasms (dystonias), hyperactivity (akathisia), and varied movements of almost any part of the body, such as the face, mouth, tongue, and arms and legs (dyskinesias). Breathing and speech can also be affected. When produced by neuroleptic drugs, the various syndromes frequently become permanent, at which point they are labeled tardive dystonia, tardive akathisia, and tardive dyskinesia.[14]

The rates for these *permanent* drug-induced disorders are astounding, probably exceeding 5 percent per year for anyone exposed for three months or more to neuroleptics. At least 25 percent of patients will become permanently afflicted after five years of exposure, and most long-term neuroleptic patients will eventually develop this irreversible adverse effect. The movements can vary in severity from barely noticeable to very severe, disfiguring, and disabling. Mental deterioration often occurs as a component.[15] In chapter 7, we will discuss the negligent attitudes of drug companies and the FDA in regard to informing the medical profession and patients about the catastrophic threat posed by tardive dyskinesia.

It now seems that Prozac can cause most of the acute,

---

*Trade names for other neuroleptics are Clozaril, Resperidol, Taractan, Inapsine, Permitil, Vesprin, Tindal, Loxitane, Serentil, Moban, Orap, Trilafon, Compazine, and Stelazine. Triavil and Etrafon contain a neuroleptic along with an antidepressant. Lithium is not a neuroleptic.

reversible neurological disorders that are also produced by the neuroleptic drugs. Prozac's pharmacological mechanism for suppressing dopamine differs from that of the neuroleptics, but clinically the result can be frighteningly similar in causing or worsening parkinsonism[16] and in producing dystonia,[17] painful neurologically induced muscle spasms. I have been told about a few cases of persistent or permanent neurological disorders from Prozac, but I have not been able to confirm them by direct examination of the patient and the history, and at present none has been reported in the literature. However, it took the profession two decades to begin to give serious attention to tardive dyskinesia, and the tendency to minimize it continues.*

Under "Adverse Reactions" of the "Nervous System," the Prozac label mentions akathisia as "infrequent," meaning it occurs in 1/100 to 1/1,000 patients. This low estimate occurs in the 1994 label despite publications estimating a vastly higher rate. It now has been established that akathisia is the most common and potentially most dangerous of the adverse neurological effects caused by Prozac. The June 1990 *Health Letter*, published by the Public Citizen Health Research Group, a Ralph Nader organization, estimates that akathisia affects a whopping 15 to 25 percent of Prozac patients.

Akathisia is characterized by inner tension or anxiety that drives or compels afflicted individuals to move their bodies. Typically the sufferer cannot sit still and frantically paces about. When severe, akathisia feels like internal torture, and those who suffer from it can wear out the soles of their shoes, the rug beneath their chair, or their clothing. It is a very common side effect in reaction to neuroleptic drugs like Haldol, Navane, Mellaril, or Thorazine, which are frequently used in the treatment of patients labeled schizophrenic, as well as the inmates and

---

*The history of professional neglect of the dangers of tardive dyskinesia is reviewed in Breggin, 1991a.

residents of prisons, nursing homes, and other institutions. Many permanent cases, called tardive akathisia, have been produced by the neuroleptics, subjecting patients to a virtual lifetime of torture.

In the September 1989 issue of the *Journal of Clinical Psychiatry,* Joseph Lipinski and his colleagues from McLean Hospital and Harvard Medical School described five cases of Prozac-induced akathisia, which they believe occurs "fairly frequently." They estimate the rate of akathisia in Prozac patients at between 9.7 percent and 25 percent. Their cases were, in their opinion, indistinguishable from neuroleptic-induced akathisia. Akathisia is frequently misdiagnosed as nervousness or agitation.

Five days after starting Prozac, one woman "reported severe anxiety and restlessness. She paced the floor throughout the day, found sleep at night difficult because of the restlessness, and constantly shifted her legs when seated." Another woman kept her roommate awake as she moved her legs so vigorously in bed it was as though she were riding a bicycle. Lipinski's group believes the effect may come from the tendency of high Prozac-induced serotonergic activity to suppress dopaminergic activity.

How could such a frequent, distressing side effect go almost wholly unrecognized among the thousands of patients tested by Eli Lilly during the FDA drug approval process? Typically, psychiatrists have tended to blame akathisia on the patient's emotional state rather than on the drugs they are being given. It's easier for doctors to invoke "mental illness" or "agitated depression" as the cause.

Meanwhile, at the request of the FDA, in March 1990 Lilly added "dyskinesia" to the list of side effects. This in no way alerts the physician to the frequency, severity, or nature of the multiple neurological disorders now associated with the drug, including the often overlooked but frequently agonizing akathisia.

Akathisia can contribute to the development of hostile or suicidal acts (chapter 6).

No permanent cases of Prozac-induced akathisia or dystonia have been reported in the literature, and I haven't personally seen any. However, no reassurance should be taken from the fact that none has been officially reported. The neuroleptics were introduced in the mid-1950s, but akathisia wasn't given credence for decades, and irreversible (tardive) akathisia and dystonia have only in the last several years become fully recognized entities.[18] In short, it's taken psychiatry more than three decades to begin to recognize the irreversibility of these drug-induced disorders.

Recently, while giving a presentation at grand rounds of a Canadian psychiatric hospital, I met a psychiatric drug expert who was hearing about tardive akathisia from a colleague for the first time. The psychiatrist was trying to blame the problem on the patient drinking too much coffee. In my experience doing consultations in North America and Europe, I find that physicians, even when they have heard of them, frequently miss the diagnoses of tardive akathisia and tardive dystonia.

Consistent with doctor denial of the dangerousness of psychiatric drugs, psychiatrists often keep patients on Prozac even after they have developed distressing neurological symptoms. Lipinski's group at Harvard, for example, continued their patients on Prozac while giving them a drug that somewhat relieved their akathisia. Despite the terrible lessons learned from the neuroleptics, they showed no concern in their report about the risk of producing permanent disorders—creating a virtual lifetime of torture in the form of tardive akathisia or tardive dystonia.

CAN PROZAC CAUSE PERMANENT NEUROTRANSMITTER ABNORMALITIES?

Prozac induces severe biochemical dysfunction in the brains of people and experimental animals, not only in the serotonergic neurotransmitter system, but in the dopaminergic and adrenergic as well. Can this dysfunction become persistent or permanent? In a sad commentary on my profession, I must state that seemingly no one, including Lilly Research Laboratories, is trying to find out. Studies of Prozac's effects almost always end shortly after the drug is stopped without testing to see if abnormalities persist for days, weeks, or months after treatment.

It's as if no one wants to know. And the FDA didn't require any such tests, although it would be *very* easy and relatively inexpensive to incorporate them into existing animal studies. First, the animal would be treated for a period of time with Prozac; next the drug would be stopped for a suitably long period of time; then the animal's brain would be examined for persistent defects, for example, in serotonergic or dopaminergic receptors. Compared to other tests performed in the Lilly laboratories, as well as in most medical centers, this is simple stuff.

As we've already seen, it can take years and even decades before psychiatrists, drug companies, or the FDA recognize obvious, frequent side effects like tardive dyskinesia, tardive akathisia, and neuroleptic malignant syndrome. But it will be even easier to overlook Prozac-induced permanent brain dysfunction, because serotonin dysfunctions do not make themselves obvious through visible symptoms, such as the twitches or spasms of tardive dyskinesia. Those neurological symptoms that have become apparent, for example, seem to result from Prozac's indirect effect on dopamine neurotransmission.

Dangerous Precedents with the Amphetamines

In their 1992 book, *Preventable Brain Damage,* Donald I. Templer, Lawrence C. Hartlage, and W. Gary Cannon discuss the difficulty of detecting serotonin dysfunction in regard to the amphetamines. Like Prozac, amphetamines block the reuptake of serotonin, and now after many years of clinical and research experience, it's been discovered that certain hallucinogenic amphetamines can permanently damage the serotonergic system.[19] One of them, MDMA ("Ecstasy") was originally considered so benign that some psychiatrists were recommending it as an adjunct to psychotherapy. In an ominous finding, when Prozac was administered along with amphetamines, it led to "greater amphetamine-induced neurotoxicity"— that is, to more drastic drug-induced malfunctions in the brain.[20]

Down-Regulation of Serotonergic Receptors

While Prozac in theory is supposed to energize the serotonin system by making more serotonin available in the synapses, in fact the brain reacts to Prozac as a toxic intrusion and tries to overcome its effects. One compensatory mechanism, called down-regulation, quickly begins reducing the number of receptors in the brain for serotonin.[21]

After being exposed to serotonin for periods of time, animal studies show that these receptors compensate by diminishing in number. The end result of down-regulation is called subsensitivity.

Down-regulation begins to occur in rats after two days of treatment with Prozac and the reductions continued over several weeks of testing, reaching up to 60 percent in some areas of the brain.* The down-regulation is widespread, involving the highest centers of the brain; for example, the frontal lobes and cortex, which regulate thinking and feeling in human beings. Down-regulation of serotonin in these areas produces complex and unpredictable effects, but is likely to reduce the capacity of the serotonin system for activation.

In chapter 7, we shall examine the implications of compensatory mechanisms for the production of abnormal behavior during Prozac treatment. Here we are concerned about the danger of permanent brain damage and dysfunction.

It has already been proven that, after months or years of treatment with other drugs, compensatory changes in receptors can become permanent, and that this can cause irreversible brain dysfunction. Tardive dyskinesia, for example, probably results from dopaminergic receptors becoming permanently hyperactive following suppression by the neuroleptic drugs.[22]

Whether Prozac's down-regulation of serotonergic receptors can become permanent remains unknown, but we must, at the very least, be very concerned about it. Unfortunately, many psychiatrists are suggesting to their patients that they should stay on Prozac for years or even for a lifetime.

PROZAC MADNESS: ADVERSE BEHAVIORAL REACTIONS

Lilly's studies for FDA approval demonstrated that Prozac can cause psychosis, especially mania. Hypomania and mania are especially disastrous reactions because they can lead people to ruin their lives, for example by risking their savings on get-rich-quick schemes, by going on shopping binges, by quitting their job or marriage, or by getting

*References in chapter 7.

involved in harebrained schemes that get them into trouble. They may engage in bizarre behavior, such as running about nude in the streets, frantically accosting cars on a busy highway, or wandering alone late at night in dangerous areas. Often the individual feels persecuted and sometimes reacts with hostility and even violence, especially toward anyone who tries to resist his or her out-of-control actions.

A typical example of Prozac-induced mania with potential violence was published by Laurence Jerome in a paper in the September 1991 issue of *The Journal of the American Academy of Child and Adolescent Psychiatry*. A ten-year-old boy became depressed when his family moved to a new neighborhood, and he was placed on 20 mgs. of Prozac by his family physician. The youngster immediately became "hyperactive, agitated," and "irritable," and his speech was pressured. He was less tired and required less sleep, and he developed a "somewhat grandiose assessment of his own abilities." Then he began to make a number of anonymous phone calls, threatening to kill a stranger in the neighborhood. When the telephone calls were traced back to him, the Prozac was discontinued and all of the hypomanic symptoms resolved within two weeks. Mania and hostility frequently go together and suggest one of the mechanisms for Prozac-induced violence, as well as for "crashing" and suicide.

Alima Jafri, M.D., and William Greenberg, M.D., from Bergen Pines County Hospital in New Jersey, describe in the September 1991 issue of the *Journal of the American Academy of Child and Adolescent Psychiatry* the case of another child who became psychotic "directly related to his receiving fluoxetine." The fifteen-year-old had become depressed after feeling rejected by his family over his disclosure of homosexuality. He was started on Prozac and the dose was increased to 40 mgs. on the fifth day, when his behavior changed:

[H]e became, in the nurses' words, very "silly," running up and down the halls teasing his peers. His running and pacing persisted, with episodes of attention-seeking crawling on the floor accompanied by animal-like growling and howling, throwing food at other adolescents, and complaining of "weird dreams." The patient reported that he felt "very good but also 'hyper,' " and admitted that he was "acting like a fool," but blamed it on his medication, which had "changed my brain." He was restless and uncharacteristically outgoing. . . .

After his medication was stopped, he improved over about one week's time.

Not all near-psychotic or psychotic reactions to Prozac have a hyper or manic quality to them. Carol Hersh and two of her physician colleagues from Cornell University Medical College in that previously cited issue of the *Journal of the Academy of Child and Adolescent Psychiatry* describe an eleven-year-old girl who developed a delusional system. The reaction occurred after only four 20-mg. doses spaced over eight days, and subsided within several days of stopping the medication.

Many other cases of relative degrees of Prozac psychosis have been published in the literature, mostly involving hypomania and mania in adults.[23] On the principle that a drug's toxic effect also explains its more subtle "therapeutic effects," many patients who swear by Prozac are probably experiencing imperceptible or barely perceptible degrees of mania. Artificial euphoria—drug-induced feelings of well-being—can be understood as an early stage of mania.

In his March 1988 report, FDA psychiatrist Kapit summarized that there were 39 reported cases of mania among the 5,620 Prozac patients in the trials. A rate of 1 percent is usually cited in the medical literature, but keep in mind that estimates made from these very short and relatively carefully monitored FDA studies are bound to demonstrate very low frequencies compared to clinical practice, especially in regard to mania. The shortness of the trials greatly limits the percentage of patients who will become affected. Early hypomanic symptoms are more likely to be spotted and nipped in the bud by stopping the medication or by adding sedative drugs. Also, there is less likelihood of Prozac being mixed with other stimulant-like drugs in the trials.

There are numerous published reports and other confirmations that Prozac can produce a variety of other mental and behavioral abnormalities, from obsessions and compulsions to murder to suicide, but these have largely been rejected or denied by both Eli Lilly and the FDA. Perhaps the most central and destructive effect of all, seen in patients like Tammy, described in an earlier chapter, is a loss of empathy for oneself and others—a kind of withdrawal from human connectedness and caring. We shall examine these tragic possibilities in later chapters.

CAN PROZAC IMPAIR THE MENTAL PROCESSES?

Under the heading of "Interference With Cognitive and Motor Performance," the Prozac label makes a general statement that "Any psychoactive drug may impair judgment, thinking, or motor skills," and it gives a warning about the use of hazardous machinery and automobiles. The label states nothing specific about Prozac itself.

Before a psychoactive drug is given to millions of people, you would think that the FDA would require testing of its effects on the mental processes, such as memory, learning, abstract reasoning, reaction time, short- and long-term memory, and so on. You would think the drug companies would be ethical enough to do it themselves, especially with a drug like Prozac that definitively affects nerves that reach into the higher mental centers of the brain.

Dozens or more studies would be necessary to begin to

explore the dangers of a drug like Prozac to higher mental functions. Even then, mental dysfunction can be too subtle to be detected on any test battery and yet profoundly affect the individual. As of 1993, two studies were available. One found no impact and the other found some memory impairment.[24]

Meanwhile, the Prozac survivors and numerous patients I have interviewed frequently report interference with memory. If you're taking Prozac, this is one more crucial area in which you are the guinea pig. The FAA doesn't let pilots take Prozac. You might consider if there isn't some wisdom in that.

SIDE EFFECTS OR PRIMARY EFFECTS?

In discussing mania, we suggested that the sought-after euphoria from Prozac can often be understood as an early stage of mania. The harmful *mental* effects of a psychiatric drug are almost always presented by psychiatrists as "side effects," as if they had nothing to do with the drug's primary or therapeutic effect. Agitation and insomnia from Prozac, for example, are seen as unrelated to its sought-after beneficial effect as an antidepressant; but they are inherent in the stimulant effect that produces feelings of energy and well-being. In this sense, the difference between "therapeutic effects" and "toxic effects" are merely steps along a continuum from mild to extreme toxicity. I have introduced this concept as the brain-disabling principle of psychiatric treatment.[25]

The neuroleptic drugs, like Haldol and Thorazine, produce a primary or therapeutic effect that consists of relative degrees of indifference or lack of interest in oneself and the environment. This is a relatively mild manifestation of the apathy caused by toxic disruption of the frontal lobes. As the doses increase, the patient becomes zombielike. These are steps along the continuum of this drug's primary toxic effect—chemical lobotomization.[26]

The comparison with sedative minor tranquilizers or alcohol is again enlightening. The person who becomes more relaxed and content after a Valium or a drink of alcohol will progress to stupor or even coma with increasing amounts. The entire experience can be understood as a spectrum of sedative toxicity.

In the case of Prozac, and all stimulant drugs, the same principle holds. At lower doses, the individual experiences signs of stimulant toxicity that may be subjectively judged as beneficial—a sense of increased alertness and energy, and a narrowing of focus and loss of emotional responsiveness. But even among patients who feel benefited, a large percentage will also suffer from nervousness or jitters, anxiety, insomnia, or loss of appetite. Even at the low dose, a significant percentage, as we've seen, will decide it's not worth taking the drug, largely because of stimulant effects. As the dose is increased, it becomes even more likely that these effects will become very uncomfortable, and at very high doses, mania and even seizures are more likely to develop.

WHEN IS A PSYCHIATRIC DRUG SAFE ENOUGH?

The analogy to alcohol and other toxic agents may once again prove helpful. Like many psychoactive drugs, alcohol has a long history of medicinal use. Even in the first half of this century, it was often prescribed by physicians as a mild and soothing sedative. Even very recently, research has suggested that small amounts of alcohol per day may reduce the risk of heart attack in males, and it's possible alcohol in very limited quantities may again be valued medicinally.

Although alcohol has been widely used throughout human society since before recorded history, only in the last decade have we begun to face the scope of its deadly impact on human behavior and society, including its association with rampant domestic violence and carnage on the highways. At the same time, we are discovering new ways in which alcohol causes illness and shortens lives. This important information is coming out after thousands of years of alcohol use and abuse by hundreds of millions of people. How, then, can we expect to evaluate our modern laboratory-tailored psychiatric drugs for safety by testing them on a few thousand people for a few brief weeks or months?

In the past few years, we have been learning more and more about the dangers of minute quantities of seemingly harmless substances in our environment. DDT, for example, was originally used lavishly in nature to kill insects, and now we have found that lingering traces of it are killing much larger animals as well. Very recent research is connecting it to breast cancer in women.[27]

While lead has been identified as a toxin for many years, it too has a fresh history as research discloses that very tiny amounts can cause brain dysfunction, behavioral abnormalities, and loss of intelligence in children.[28]

When psychiatric drugs like Prozac are introduced into the brain, their concentrations are infinitely higher than toxic exposures within the larger, natural environment from substances like lead or DDT. If we can cause such damage to ourselves and to our world with relatively minuscule toxic additives to the physical universe, imagine what we must be doing when we pour far higher concentrations of pollutants into our more delicate and sensitive brains. And remember, the psychiatric drugs are specifically designed to interfere with normal biological processes like neurotransmission. We can only begin to guess at the long-term negative consequences and may never fully be able to grasp them.

HARMONIZING NEUROTRANSMITTERS OR DISABLING THE BRAIN?

Prozac and the other SSRIs turn out to be no different than any other physical intervention in psychiatry: there's no qualitative difference between the therapeutic and the toxic effect; it's a matter of degree. Whether or not the individual feels better, the brain has suffered a disruptive intrusion. The greater the mental impact of the drug, the greater the disability that's been imposed upon the brain.

In psychiatry, the tendency is to deny this seemingly obvious truth. As psychiatrists, we like to imagine that we are instead doing something good to the brain and even improving its function by correcting imbalances or harmonizing neurotransmitters. This argument in recent years has been made with equal zeal for shock treatment. Like Prozac, shock treatment is alleged to work by enhancing serotonin[29]—even though the shocked brain is so grossly traumatized that the patient is rendered too confused and blunted to feel any subtle emotions. Even brain-mutilating lobotomy is nowadays justified on the grounds that it corrects biochemical imbalances, and one advocate looks forward to delivering serotonin "psychosurgically" to "serotonin-depleted sites" in the brain.[30]

And so Prozac is said to "enhance" serotonergic neurotransmission when in fact it grossly impairs the process of neurotransmission. We know about the impairment—we can measure the blocking of the normal reuptake process, as well as the brain's attempts to compensate with various mechanisms.* Prozac creates this havoc in any person, as well as in rats with normal brains.

We can only speculate about the alleged improvement—that somehow it's better to interfere in this way in the brain's normal processes. Psychiatry must overcome

---

*Other ominous changes will be discussed in chapters 5–7.

scientific fact with rhetoric in order to claim that this drug improves the functioning of anyone's brain.

The argument that Prozac somehow corrects an imbalance—surely a lucky stroke if it sometimes happens—makes much less sense than the proven observation that it botches up normal processes. On the face of it, how could a pill produce such fine tuning? It doesn't have the sophistication or technology to do so. All the pill can do is to make a massive intervention and hope for the best. It is, after all, only a pill. It has no built-in capacity to evaluate the situation and to make the necessary adjustments, while the brain is in fact sizing up the situation, and trying to mute the drug effect. Meanwhile, the physician, adjusting the dose from week to week or month to month, is in no better position. At best, he's grossly monitoring and adjusting levels of drug toxicity, while the brain tries mightily to resist the effort.

The physician who gives Prozac is not comparable to a highly skilled mechanic using computerized technology to fuss over your relatively simple automobile engine. He's more like a clumsy office colleague spilling his coffee into your computer—except Prozac is much more potent than caffeine and your brain is far more vulnerable and easily damaged than your computer.

Taking Prozac, in sum, constitutes a toxic interference into the brain. If it feels good, it means that the individual prefers impaired brain function to normal brain function. That some people prefer stimulant intoxication and some people sedatives, or that some people like a mixture, should not distract us from the basic principle.

The desire for an impaired brain is not an unusual preference in Western society. Given the complexity and difficulty of modern life, as well as our lack of preparation for it, it's readily understandable that people sometimes prefer a toxic state. Most people have been tempted at one time or another by cigarettes, coffee, alcohol, or a variety of illicit drugs, and many struggle compulsively with these agents. We should try, as this book title suggests, to talk back to and to resist these temptations.

As in drinking alcohol, the choice should be up to the individual. But psychiatry and the drug companies should not mislead the public and patients into thinking that something more benign is going on. It is our hope that this chapter will make you more aware that doctors, drug companies, and even the FDA may not always have your best interests at heart, and that Prozac's label does not tell the whole story about the very real and potentially devastating side effects of this drug.

Meanwhile, if you have suffered a serious adverse reaction to Prozac, Paxil, or Zoloft (or any other medication), you or your physician can send an adverse reaction report directly to the FDA. The FDA's new reporting form is replicated in the Appendix.

We turn now to one particular hazard that deserves special attention: the possibility of withdrawal symptoms, addiction, and abuse associated with Prozac.

FIVE

Drug Addiction and Abuse

A Comparison Between Prozac and Amphetamines

Drug addiction is the inability to resist or break the habit of taking a psychoactive drug. In severe cases, it can lead to criminal behavior, ill health, and the overall deterioration of the quality of life. Addiction may be driven by psychological needs, as well as by physiological craving created by the drug itself.

Drug abuse is the use of any psychoactive drug in a compulsive or pleasure-seeking manner that results in harmful effects. People who abuse drugs frequently become addicted.

Drugs associated with addiction and abuse usually cause withdrawal symptoms. The addiction and abuse, however, are typically driven by the individual's craving for the positive effects produced by the drug rather than by fear of going through a painful withdrawal. Addictive drugs tend to provide pleasure, a sense of energy or euphoria, or a sedative (tranquilizing) escape from painful emotions, such as anxiety and tension.

Withdrawal from certain drugs can produce obvious and even life-threatening symptoms. Abruptly stopping the use of large amounts of alcohol or sedatives, including minor tranquilizers, can produce seizures or cardiovascular collapse. But withdrawal from stimulant drugs, such as amphetamines and cocaine, does not produce physically dangerous symptoms. Withdrawal from them, instead, tends to cause mental pain, often in the form of extreme fatigue and depression, and even suicidal impulses. Users of stimulants end up feeling that they cannot go on living without their drugs.

That people often return to addictive drugs years after stopping them suggests that they are mainly seeking the drug's positive effects. On the other hand, the long-term craving may itself be an attenuated, persistent withdrawal response.

Without deriving any positive feelings from psychiatric drug usage, some patients feel compelled to keep taking them out of fear of the psychological consequences of stopping them. I often treat people who seem to derive little or no benefit, and no pleasure, from one Prozac or one Klonopin per day, but who remain afraid to give up the drug. When they try to stop, they become anxious and afraid even before physical withdrawal can take place.

While drug addicts and abusers often feel their lives are immeasurably enhanced by drugs, their judgment often seems questionable. The user may feel "better than ever," but more objective observers may conclude that this feeling is illusory. The positive effects of these drugs are often temporary or destined to change into negative ones.

Drug addicts and abusers do not necessarily escalate the dosage of drug. Many people are addicted to legal drugs such as nicotine, caffeine, or alcohol for most of their lives without significantly increasing the amount of their intake over time. The same is true of many individuals who use illegal drugs, such as marijuana, or nonprescription opiates and amphetamines. The chronic use of the drugs at relatively constant doses can, however, result in negative physical and psychological effects.

DARVON: A SKELETON IN ELI LILLY'S CLOSET

Eli Lilly and the FDA take the position, as expressed in the Prozac label, that Prozac-induced dependence, abuse, and withdrawal have not been demonstrated. The Prozac label does, however, acknowledge that its testing "was not systematic" in this regard and "it is not possible to predict on the basis of this limited experience the extent to which a CNS [central nervous system] active drug will be misused, diverted, and/or abused once marketed."

Drug companies, doctors, and the FDA have typically been remiss in recognizing the addictive or habit-forming qualities of prescription medications, as well as the withdrawal problems.* In *The Tranquilizing of America,* reporters Richard Hughes and Robert Brewin compare pharmaceutical company promotion of drugs to "the patent-medicine men who once roamed this country with horse and wagon, huckstering magic elixirs to naive audiences." They go on to indict Eli Lilly for its promotion of Darvon (propoxyphene):

> As an example of this kind of selling and the success drug companies have is the campaign for Darvon, the painkiller that now tops the nation's legal drug death list.† Lilly introduced Darvon in 1957 with much fanfare, promoting it via magazine advertisements and detail men as a potent painkiller without the potential for abuse and addiction shown by earlier painkillers, such as codeine. The company's ads and the detail men constantly emphasized that Darvon was a nonnarcotic and therefore nonaddicting analgesic.

Lilly's persistent denials of any addictive or life-threatening dangers from Darvon were especially extraordinary in light of its chemical similarity to another well-known narcotic, methadone. A glance from even the untutored eye discloses that their chemical structures are nearly identical[1] and modern pharmacology classifies Dar-

---

*Valium (diazepam) and other minor tranquilizers, for example, were supposed to be less addictive and to have fewer withdrawal symptoms than earlier sedatives, but this turned out to be untrue.

†With more cautious use of the drug, this is no longer so.

von with methadone, meperidine (Demerol), and codeine. Yet for years, Lilly's FDA-monitored promotional materials denied any addiction problems from Darvon. The 1963 *Physicians' Desk Reference (PDR)*, for example, states outright that Darvon "does not have characteristics that would lead to abuse of the drug and to addiction."

Twenty years after Darvon came into use, the Department of Justice reported that it was widely abused as an addictive drug and should be classified as a narcotic. In 1977, Lilly continued to prosper from Darvon, which earned $140 million in revenues, as it became the third best-selling prescription drug in America. At the same time, Darvon became the second most frequently mentioned drug in coroner's reports, only behind heroin in its association with drug-related deaths.

In 1978 Ralph Nader's Health Research Group petitioned the government to have Darvon banned, but Lilly did not let up its sales efforts, even as the U.S. Senate held hearings.[2] During the buildup of the controversy, Lilly's promotional material, as illustrated by the *PDR*, did acknowledge "drug dependence characterized by psychic dependence and, less frequently, physical dependence and tolerance," and compared the problems to that of codeine. The statement, however, was relatively lost in the text.

Finally in 1980, more than two decades after the drug was first marketed to the public, the FDA required Lilly to display a large box in its promotional materials. Nearly one column deep, it is headlined "WARNINGS." The text in the box, with a bullet and bold print, begins "Do not prescribe [Darvon] for patients who are suicidal or addiction-prone."

Neither the pharmaceutical companies nor the FDA can be relied upon to protect America from even the most dangerous adverse effects of psychoactive drugs before they cause havoc.

PARALLELS BETWEEN PROZAC AND THE CLASSIC STIMULANTS

Since the SSRIs, including Prozac, have a stimulant profile of effects, it is useful to compare them to the classic stimulants, such as amphetamines and cocaine, in regard to their potential for addiction, abuse, and withdrawal symptoms.

Listening to Cocaine

Early in the sixteenth century, the Spanish *conquistadores* encountered the empire of the Incas and found them using the coca leaf in their religious rituals.[3] European interest in the medicinal qualities of coca leaf grew slowly in the mid-nineteenth century. By 1878 advertisements in the United States promoted it for "young persons afflicted with timidity in society." In 1883 the American manufacturer Parke-Davis advertised it in medical journals as a treatment for morphine addiction and alcoholism.

Cocaine was first isolated from the coca plant in Germany in 1882. In 1883 a German army physician, Theodor Aschenbrandt, gave it to Bavarian soldiers on maneuvers and found that it improved their ability to surmount fatigue. Twenty-eight-year-old Sigmund Freud read Aschenbrandt's account and procured an amount for experimentation on his own patients and tried some himself.[4]

A poverty-ridden, professionally frustrated young man who suffered from periodic depression and exhaustion, Freud immediately became more cheerful after taking cocaine. He proclaimed it a "miracle drug" and in 1884 wrote to his fiancée, Martha Bernays, that he'd begun to take "small doses of it regularly against depression and

against indigestion, and with the most brilliant success."
He told her, "In my last severe depression I took coca
again and a small dose lifted me to the heights in a wonderful fashion. I am just now busy collecting the literature
for a song of praise to this magical substance." He sent
some to Martha for her own use.

In three months or less, Freud published an article ex-
tolling cocaine. His essay, according to biographer Ernest
Jones, was written in the most brilliant style Freud would
ever achieve. Jones observed, "There is, moreover, in this
essay a tone that never recurred in Freud's writings, a
remarkable combination of objectivity with a personal
warmth as if he were in love with the content itself." Out
of style for a scientific essay, Freud referred to administering an "offering" instead of a "dose" and used expressions such as "the most gorgeous excitement" to
describe cocaine's effects. All this becomes even more remarkable in the light of Freud's seemingly loveless and
cynical attitude toward most things in life, including people in general.

In language uncannily similar to that of many of the
Prozac users described in Peter Kramer's *Listening to
Prozac,* Freud wrote that cocaine produced:

> [E]xhilaration and lasting euphoria, which in no way dif-
> fers from the normal euphoria of the healthy person. . . .
> You perceive an increase of self-control and possess more
> vitality and capacity for work. . . . In other words, you are
> simply normal, and it is soon hard to believe that you
> are under the influence of any drug. . . . Long intensive
> mental or physical work is performed without fatigue. . . .
> The result is enjoyed without any of the unpleasant after-
> effects that follow exhilaration brought about by alco-
> hol. . . . Absolutely no craving for the further use of co-
> caine appears after the first, or even after repeated taking
> of the drug; one feels rather a certain curious aversion to
> it. [Ellipses in Jones, 1953]

Freud experimented with cocaine for approximately three years before its dangers made him give it up. In the process, he came under medical criticism for encouraging the use of such an addictive and mentally disabling substance.

By 1890 the dangers of cocaine were widely known, but it continued to be used in popular drinks and various tonics, including those for shrinking the nasal membranes. Then in 1914, cocaine was subjected to the same controls as those for morphine and heroin, and state laws began to identify it as a "narcotic." It is no longer used in psychiatry but has limited medical application as a surface or skin anesthetic.

Listening to Amphetamine

The first amphetamine was synthesized in 1887, but its stimulant properties were not recognized for forty years. Beginning with amphetamine (Benzedrine) in 1936 and later with dextroamphetamine (Dexedrine), these lab-produced drugs helped to usher in the modern era of antidepressants. Later on, methamphetamine (Methedrine, Desoxyn) became widely used as a potent street drug. Methylphenidate (Ritalin) is an amphetamine-like drug with essentially the same pharmacological properties.

In language that once again anticipates today's claims for Prozac, medical reports in the 1930s made claims for startling emotional transformations in many or most patients receiving amphetamines. One researcher spoke of the "immediate, and often dramatic, value in breaking the stranglehold of depression, restoring 'energy feeling,' and renewing optimism, self-assurance, increased initiative, appetite for work, and zest for living."[5]

At a 1970 conference on amphetamines sponsored by the National Institute of Mental Health (NIMH),[6] Roger Smith from the Department of Pharmacology at the University of California described how the desired effects of speed include increased feelings of "confidence and well-being" and increased ability to perform motor tasks. Some users view speed as a consciousness-expanding drug. They find speed enables them to overcome their inhibitions and, in the words of one user, to "think and rap and get all of my philosophies out."

In a similar vein, Everett Ellinwood, Jr., of the department of psychiatry at Duke described how users initially display "loquaciousness, decreased ambivalence, a sense of cleverness and crystal-clear thinking, and an invigorating aggressiveness." Another expert, John C. Kramer, verified that the drug produced "the feeling of ability and of invulnerability." "Suddenly, magically, volubility and gregariousness appear and boredom departs."

A 1972 Consumers Union Report quoted expert Roger Smith:

> Many of the young people who are currently involved in the speed scene report that they were initially attracted to the drug because of the instant improvement noted in self-image. Many suffered from feelings of inferiority and lack of self-worth, which manifested itself in chronic, and often debilitating, depression.

Smith observed that creativity seemed at times to be enhanced. In the Haight-Ashbury speed culture of the 1960s, one woman compulsively drove herself to learn to play the guitar, practicing until her fingers were cut and bleeding. But she did learn and retain the skill. "Several artists changed their styles completely after turning to speed. Many began working with pen and ink, producing drawings of great detail and complexity."

There is nothing unique about "listening to Prozac." People were "listening to speed" in much the same way, and in even greater numbers, in the 1960s.

Amphetamines and SSRIS: Prescribed for Nearly Identical Purposes

Prescriptions for amphetamines, like those for the SSRIs, were written for depression, fatigue, and anxiety, as well as obesity. They were also prescribed for "facilitation of psychotherapy." Smith Kline and French advertised Dexamyl Spansules (a combination of Dexedrine and a sedative) in the September 8, 1955, *New England Journal of Medicine* as a miraculous panacea:

> *For day-long relief of anxiety and depression in*:
> Premenstrual tension
> Menopausal depression
> Chronic headache and backache
> Bronchial asthma
> Abdominal spasm
> Alcoholism
> Convalescence
> Arthritis
> Weakness and vertigo
> Pain or inactivity of chronic disease
> Obesity
> Psychogenic fatigue.

The ad promised that one daily dose of the long-acting preparation gives continuous all-day "relief of the mental and emotional distress you see in almost every patient." The blanket claim for success and the wide spectrum of recommended applications bears a shocking resemblance to professional and public attitudes toward Prozac.

The legalized amphetamine craze vastly exceeded that as yet achieved by Prozac and the other SSRIs. Mitchell Balter of the National Institute of Mental Health[7] estimated that approximately 12 million adults in the United States—6 to 8 percent of the total population—used amphetamines by prescription in 1967. Druggists filled 23.3 million prescriptions for amphetamines, alone or in combination, in that year—approximately double the current rate for Prozac. This comprised 14 percent of all psychoactive drug prescriptions sold in the United States. About 80 percent of the patients were women.

Despite the enormous enthusiasm that persisted for decades, Benzedrine was eventually withdrawn from the market because of its side effects and lack of efficacy, and last appeared in the 1982 *PDR*. The extremely popular combinations of amphetamines with sedatives were also withdrawn by the FDA, and Dexamyl last appeared in the 1980 *PDR*.

Dexedrine has remained available, but in the 1970s Smith Kline and French was required to limit substantially its therapeutic claims. Once a "miracle" drug for depression, the FDA expunged depression from its list of officially sanctioned uses. The amphetamine is now approved only for narcolepsy (uncontrollable episodes of falling asleep) and attention deficit disorder with hyperactivity.

Once regarded "as versatile remedies that were second only to a few other extraordinary drugs like aspirin in the scope, efficacy, and safety," amphetamines are currently viewed with grave caution.[8] The similarity of their effects and side effects to those of the SSRIs suggests caution about Prozac, Zoloft, and Paxil.

Amphetamine and SSRI Withdrawal

The medical profession and the public can be misled by the idea that addiction must involve obvious symptoms of physical withdrawal, such as nausea and vomiting, seizures, or cardiovascular collapse, none of which tend to occur with cocaine, the amphetamines, or SSRIs. The *DSM-III-R* confirms that in amphetamine withdrawal, "Paranoid and suicidal ideation [thoughts] may be present" and "Suicide is the major complication."

In my workshops and consultations, I have become familiar with many cases of SSRI withdrawal, usually in the form of "crashing" with depression and fatigue, frequently accompanied by suicidal impulses. One woman in my practice with mild depression was being prescribed Zoloft by another physician. She spontaneously decided to reduce her Zoloft from 100 mgs. to 50 mgs. per day, and within a day or two lapsed into exhaustion and fatigue, profound depression, and a compulsive, alien-feeling desire to kill herself that seemed unrelated to any circumstances in her life. She felt improved, with complete relief from the suicidal feelings, soon after resuming the 100-mg. dose. She asked me to take over her medication treatment and, with careful supervision and the involvement of a close friend who lived with her, she tapered off the drug in one week. I had wanted her to take somewhat longer, but she was already feeling much better after six or seven days, and completely better in another week or two.

In the case of Catherine, which I published in the medical literature,[9] I gave a consultation to a young woman who was prescribed Prozac for depression associated with the recollection of verified childhood sexual abuse. When out of town one weekend, she forgot to bring along her Prozac, and became "frantic to get it." She risked embarrassment by asking acquaintances at a conference if they knew people who might share their Prozac with her, and was relieved when someone volunteered. When she accidentally skipped her Prozac on one other occasion, her co-workers noticed her listlessly moping about and asked if she'd forgotten her medication. She did not, however, feel a craving to take more than her regular dose.

Initially Catherine felt energized by Prozac and her depression was only partially relieved. Later in treatment, she became more severely depressed and suicidal for the first time since the actual abuse during childhood. An increase of Prozac to 40 mgs. did not relieve her depression, which led to her psychiatric hospitalization. She refused further medication and the depression gradually abated after termination of the Prozac. Her depression was probably drug-induced, caused by the reaction of her brain against the Prozac.

Physicians Alan Louie, Richard Lannon, and Luriko Ajari published in the March 1994 *American Journal of Psychiatry* a case of withdrawal from Zoloft involving "fatigue, severe abdominal cramps, and distention" as well as "insomnia, increased dreaming, slight shortness of breath, impairment of short-term memory, and influenza-like symptoms consisting of general aching, chills without fever, headache, and sore eyes." All these symptoms quickly abated when Zoloft was restarted at a small dose. The authors believe that withdrawal may turn out to be more common with Zoloft than with Prozac because of the former's shorter half-life. They believe the withdrawal may also be due to Zoloft's capacity to affect two other receptor systems, acetylcholine and the opioids.

Amphetamine and Prozac Drug Abuse

The dangers of amphetamine abuse and addiction were first reported in the medical literature by E. Guttman as early as 1939, a mere two years after Benzedrine was synthesized. But relatively few voices were raised in concern and it would be decades before official recognition of the dangers.

The 1957 World Health Organization (WHO) report on amphetamine addiction commented that abusers ingest "amounts far exceeding the usual therapeutic dose, they may be prepared to break the law to obtain supplies, they are dependent upon it, and sometimes become psychotic. Furthermore, withdrawal symptoms may occur, notably states of depression in which suicide may occur."[10]

The illicit abuse of amphetamines broke out in epidemics, as in Japan in 1954–6, Scandinavia in 1965–8, and California's Haight-Ashbury in 1966–9. Many of the reports we have drawn upon in this chapter came from expertise developed as a result of the Haight-Ashbury experience.

In 1975 Grinspoon and Hedblom pointed out that withdrawal problems can occur "when amphetamine has been taken only for a short time and the dosage has not been increased," but that it is most severe after the user has been taking high, intravenous doses. In 1975 Grinspoon and Hedblom declared, "Contrary to much medical and popular opinion, the amphetamines are probably as addictive as heroin."

Any routine use of stimulants for managing life is likely to be harmful. In the 1966 *Journal of the American Medical Association,* P. H. Connell, M.D., described the various levels of amphetamine dependence among adolescents, and pointed out that even relying on two or three tablets per day was injurious.

By the 1960s, in part through awareness of massive drug abuse in the Haight-Ashbury section of San Francisco, many experts became convinced about amphetamine's potential for serious abuse. But as the large numbers of prescriptions at the time indicate, practicing physicians, some of the medical establishment, and the pharmaceutical industry were slow to recognize the seriousness of these problems.

In the 1960s, the *Physicians' Desk Reference* began to recognize that there was a danger of "psychological dependence," but only in "unstable individuals." It was not until 1975—after nearly forty-five years of clinical use—that the FDA finally required Smith Kline and French to place a separate box in the *PDR* that warns in capitalized letters that amphetamines "have a high potential for abuse." The FDA and the drug companies listed "assaultiveness" under overdose, but never acknowledged the widespread problem of paranoid ideation and violence, including murder. The latest 1994 *PDR*, with its FDA-approved description of the drug, persists in this failure to underscore the danger of violence and there is still no mention of suicide.

The history of the pharmaceutical industry and the FDA in regard to amphetamines is telling. Similarly, the evidence is mounting in regard to Prozac-induced abuse, violence, and suicide. One wonders how long it will take the FDA and industry to give official recognition to the dangers posed by Prozac. Meanwhile, evidence is building for Prozac abuse.

Marcus Goldman, Lester Grinspoon, and Susan Hunter-Jones mention anecdotal reports from Italy that indicate a new "illicit" drug known as "Bye-Bye Blues" is in fact Prozac. The authors describe their own case of a former drug abuser who claimed to achieve a high on Prozac from as little as 1 mg. per day. After breaking open the capsule, "She ingested the powder by sucking it into her mouth and described the experience as similar to 'speeding'—giving her increased energy and the ability to interact socially with others." Much as any speed addict, she titrated her dose to balance between excessive stimulation and severe drowsiness. James Wilcox reported a case of "abuse" concerning an anorectic woman who took up to 120 mgs. per day in a successful effort to lose weight.

We have recently heard anecdotal stories of college students sniffing Prozac for a high. High school students who formerly abused drugs have informed us that there is a great deal of experimentation with Prozac. Youngsters are trying to snort and to smoke it. Whether it produces a real high under these conditions seemed uncertain to our informants. They are aware of occasional individuals who do get high by ingesting Prozac and who try to obtain it from doctors for that purpose.

One of my patients was asked by his fourteen-year-old son if he could get some Prozac. There were other boys in class who were glad to be taking Prozac because it made them feel good and some of them had been passing it around. When children start asking for a drug, it's a sign that abuse is possible.

The street value of Prozac among youngsters in Bethesda, Maryland, we are told by former drug abusers, is

$3 to $4 per pill. The price remains relatively low because the drug is so readily available to youngsters through their own psychiatrists and pediatricians.

EVIDENCE FROM THE STREETS ABOUT PROZAC'S POTENTIAL FOR ABUSE AND ADDICTION

In a retrospective on the synthesis of amphetamines in his laboratory years earlier, Chauncey Leake commented on his dismay when these stimulants began to be abused during the 1960s in California:

> It was shocking to learn in connection with the drug culture in the Haight-Ashbury district of San Francisco, that methamphetamine was beginning to be obtained on the black market, and used by vein. This is certainly something we never anticipated. It was badly abused.

Is the same story unfolding once again in the same place—Haight-Ashbury—this time with Prozac?

Darryl Inaba is a doctor of pharmacy who, since 1967, has worked in the Haight-Ashbury Free Clinic, where he is now director of drug-abuse treatment programs. My attention was drawn to Inaba through an interview entitled "Prozac 'Abuse'" by Fred Gardner in the *Anderson Valley Advertiser* (California). Inaba told Gardner "from its early use in our clinical situation, patients mentioned that it had an arousal effect. . . . Prozac offered you actual, perceivable good feelings. Creative, reinforcing, positive. . . ."

Inaba and his colleagues were originally attracted by the margin of safety in regard to suicide. But then:

> We got concerned about the very pleasurable, reinforcing arousal effect, because we're dealing with a population that likes to be in pleasure, and may misuse any drug that brings them pleasure. We've had some testimonies from

clients who claim they inject Prozac, and others who take it to get high. . . . A lot of people are taking Prozac now and claiming they're "better than normal." That's a scary phrase. What is "better than normal"?

As a doctor of pharmacy, Inaba was able to comment on Effexor, a drug that blocks the reuptake of both serotonin and norepinephrine. He observed, "Well, they're getting pretty close to cocaine and speed there." Cocaine and amphetamine block the reuptake of serotonin and norepinephrine, and also dopamine.

Inaba expressed concern about the possibility of unsuspected long-term damaging effects from SSRIs: "Despite the hurdles and hoops that the FDA makes people go through to get a drug approved, we still end up with a guinea pig situation."

I interviewed Inaba by telephone on March 14 of this year. He confirmed his interview with Gardner and explained that his group of addiction-prone patients were especially sensitive to any drug's abuse potential. To date, Inaba has seen about a dozen cases of Prozac abuse, including injecting the drug or getting high on the capsules. Included in the dozen are individuals who had kicked their speed or cocaine habit, only to have it restimulated by taking Prozac. Prozac became a transition drug back to addiction and abuse.

The current "casual" attitude toward Prozac reminds Inaba of Valium during the 1960s and 1970s. Like Prozac, it was promoted as nonaddictive and also as relatively safe in overdose. Yet Valium turned out to be addictive and to be very dangerous in overdose when combined with other drugs and alcohol.

There seems no doubt that Prozac abuse has begun. How far it will escalate remains to be seen.

RESEARCH EVIDENCE FOR PROZAC'S ABUSE POTENTIAL

If Prozac has an abuse potential similar to that of the stimulants, then laboratory studies should be able to demonstrate that Prozac can actually substitute for stimulants in animals who have been trained to use them. Specifically, will animals find the craving for amphetamines relieved by Prozac?

Linda Porrino and a team at the National Institute of Neurological Diseases and Stroke reviewed the literature and observed that animals want less amphetamine when given drugs such as Prozac that stimulate serotonergic nerves. Porrino's own study found that pre-treatment with Prozac reduced a rat's desire for amphetamine. While she raises doubts about the hypothesis, she recognizes that her data suggest that Prozac "may be potentiating the effects of or substituting for amphetamine." Similarly, Dianna Yu and a team from the Texas Tech University Health Sciences Center reported that injections of Prozac into rats markedly reduced their intake of amphetamine.[11]

Can the same phenomenon be demonstrated in experiments with humans? As indicated by Inaba's report from the Haight-Ashbury clinic, will people substitute Prozac for stimulants and vice versa?

In the February 1993 *Psychiatric Times,* Yale professor of psychiatry Thomas Kosten cites two as-yet-unpublished studies confirming the Prozac-cocaine connection. One shows that Prozac can significantly reduce cocaine abuse in patients, while another, by Kosten himself, has shown that Zoloft can ameliorate cocaine abuse.

In a published research project, psychiatrists Mark Pollack and Jerrold Rosenbaum of the Massachusetts General Hospital administered Prozac to eleven cocaine abusers, five of whom were successfully treated. Pollack and Rosenbaum present case examples in which Prozac relieved the "craving" for cocaine, enabling the patients to abstain from the stimulant while taking the SSRI. Other studies have failed to confirm these positive results, and it will take a while to determine how interchangeable Prozac is with stimulants.

In comparing Prozac, Zoloft, or Paxil to speed, it is generally true that comparable psychoactive drugs that have more immediate and short-lived effects will have a more profoundly disruptive effect on the brain and mind.

Prozac and the other SSRIs usually—but not always—require several doses to have a noticeable impact on the individual. The buildup to maximum effect can take ten days to four weeks. By contrast, cocaine and amphetamine both take effect rapidly, sometimes within minutes. Some methods of using crack cocaine are nearly instantaneous—causing a dramatic high.

The SSRIs, slower to get started, are also slower to wear off. Prozac, for example, remains at half its original concentration in the bloodstream for up to nine or ten days after stopping the drug, and can continue to have an effect long afterward. The half-life of Zoloft's major active metabolite is much less, in the range of 62 to 104 hours. The half-life for Paxil is yet shorter, in the range of one day, but still much longer than that of the classical stimulants.

Because of their relatively short half-lives, we would expect greater withdrawal reactions for Zoloft and especially Paxil, and as we already described, there is a recent case of withdrawal reaction from Zoloft reported in the literature.[12] While withdrawal reactions play only a part in the addiction syndrome, they often signal that a drug has abuse potential.

In sharp contrast to all of the current SSRIs, Dexedrine's concentration in the blood is halved in half a day, while Ritalin's is halved in a mere three hours or so after the last dose. Cocaine's loss of effect is even more rapid, depending on the method of administration.

The difference in rapidity of onset and length of duration means that Prozac will tend to have a smoother action than the other SSRIs and the classical stimulants. Cocaine and amphetamines more drastically jerk the brain up and down with their abrupt onset and quick washout. To the extent that Prozac mimics speed as a stimulant drug, it will do so less dramatically in most cases. But over time, the effect may be no less dramatic or disastrous.

PETER KRAMER AND THE PROZAC-COCAINE CONNECTION

After toying with the question throughout *Listening to Prozac,* Peter Kramer concludes that a fine distinction can be drawn between Prozac and stimulants like cocaine: "Prozac simply gives anhedonic [lacking in pleasure] people access to pleasures identical to those enjoyed by other normal people in their ordinary social pursuits."[13] In other words, a Prozac "high" isn't really high—it's normal.

But how can Kramer distinguish between an abnormal drug-induced high and a normal drug-induced mood elevation? We shall repeatedly find that Prozac mood elevation can come at the expense of sensitivity—a fact that Kramer himself stresses. And, further, it can come at the expense of rationality and judgment. On the other hand, it's also apparent that Kramer's claim—that Prozac promotes *normal* zest—is precisely what most users of stimulants have always claimed, from Sigmund Freud in nineteenth-century Europe to youngsters snorting and inhaling the same substance in contemporary America.

Kramer also justifies Prozac by exaggerating the addictive qualities of amphetamines and cocaine: "Cocaine and amphetamine do not satiate but, rather, excite further desire; stimulant addicts will tend to 'go on a run' and rapidly use all the drug at their disposal."[14] While this is true of some desperate addicts, the vast majority of stimulant users do not respond in this manner, especially when the drug is prescribed by a physician. For example, amphetamines, including Ritalin, are now routinely administered to children and adults diagnosed with Attention Deficit–Hyperactivity Disorder (ADHD), with only a relatively small percentage of people escalating their dosages. Yet amphetamines are recognized as highly addictive.

Similarly, Kramer states that, "Amphetamines, cocaine, heroin, opium, alcohol, and other street drugs used to elevate mood all ultimately result in a 'crash.' " But such a blanket statement is untrue. Millions of people have used those addictive drugs—including opium and alcohol—often for a lifetime, while remaining on a relatively even emotional keel.

Speaking of one of his own cases in a similar vein, Kramer says, "Hillary's initial short-lived success on Prozac sounds like a favorable reaction to 'amphetaminelike effect,' except that it lasted weeks rather than days."[15] Kramer's emphasis is incorrect. As Freud initially found, cocaine—as well as most stimulants—can maintain its impact after months or years of use. Millions of people use prescribed and illicit stimulants, from caffeine to cocaine, for years on end without losing the drug effect. And while the effect does tend to wear off for some people who use classic stimulants, it also wears off for some people who use SSRIs.

To this day, many physicians continue to underestimate the dangers of amphetamines, much as they miscalculate the problems associated with Prozac. Under the Controlled Substances Act, the FDA classifies Ritalin in Schedule II—the most addictive class of drugs in medical use. It shares Schedule II with other stimulants (Dexedrine and cocaine) and with narcotics (morphine).[16] This places it two categories above the minor tranquilizers, like Valium and Xanax, in terms of degree of addictive potential. Yet doctors who prescribe Ritalin for children routinely overlook the fact that it is a form of "speed." They tell patients and their families that it is not habit forming. CH.A.D.D. (Children with Attention Deficit Disorders), a parents' organization that favors drugging their children with Ritalin, is currently lobbying the FDA to remove Ritalin from Schedule II.

We turn now to a yet more menacing connection between SSRIs, such as Prozac, and amphetamines—the production of violence and suicide.

SIX

Drug-Induced Paranoia, Violence, Depression, and Suicide

A Comparison Between Prozac and Amphetamines

At six-foot-two-inches with a trim build, blue eyes, and golden hair, thirty-seven-year-old Dwight Harlor III looks like a grown-up boy scout. If he weren't shy, he'd come across like a movie star.

Most of Dwight's life has been as unblemished as his appearance. Until recently, he had no history of psychiatric problems, let alone suicidal or homicidal tendencies. Two speeding tickets in a lifetime comprised his brushes with the law. He's a conservative midwesterner.

In the fall of 1989 stresses began to build in Dwight's family life. His mother had a series of strokes that resulted in a coma. After she awoke, she was never again able to take care of herself. A few months later, Dwight's father suffered a heart attack and required surgery, and Dwight and his wife found themselves nursing both his parents. According to Dwight, these and additional stresses in his wife's family were too much for them to weather as a couple, and his wife separated from him and obtained a divorce in January 1991.*

Dwight had ongoing, acrimonious conflicts with his estranged and then former wife. He felt betrayed and could not bear losing her. On one occasion prior to their sepa-

---

*Since I'm not disguising Dwight's identity, I won't go into the details of his conflicts with his wife, but there was no history of violence.

ration, he shook her and gave her a vague warning during an argument. He did have a temper and would at times yell at her, but beyond the incident of shaking her, he never threatened or perpetrated violence.

At the time of the divorce, Dwight was employed as a quality-control engineer at an aircraft company, and he continued to perform well at work. Among thirty-two employees in 1990, he was one of two who received a superior rating. He was well liked on the job and was viewed as a very friendly, cooperative, genuine, and intelligent man. His previous work record was good, too, and he'd been given a high security clearance.

During the illnesses of his parents and then the divorce, Dwight became increasingly upset and depressed, although he was never suicidal, and his work remained unimpaired. The nurse at the company clinic suggested Prozac and referred Dwight to a general practitioner as well as to a psychotherapist. At the end of August 1990, Dwight started taking 20 mgs. of Prozac each morning by prescription from his general practitioner, and in a few days he felt much better. He reports, "It gave me energy, made me cheerful, and gave me the desire to get out and do things." Not one to rely on others for help, Dwight attended only a few therapy sessions. Besides, Prozac was all he needed.

Dwight was unaware of most of the changes taking place in him after he started Prozac, and could not fully describe what happened to his work relationships; but co-workers and friends, who did not know he was taking a psychiatric medication, saw him transform into a totally different person. According to a man who knew Dwight well, over a two-month period Dwight grew increasingly "hyper," impatient, belligerent, and difficult to work with. He would become outraged in meetings and retreat into his office and cry. His memory, usually very sharp, seemed to be failing him, and he became forgetful.

Another of Dwight's co-workers, an engineer whose former boyfriend had used amphetamines, wondered if

Dwight was taking speed. When she tried to ask Dwight about it, he wouldn't tell her anything about the pills he was taking except "I need them." She told me, "He sounded hooked." She was not surprised when another concerned colleague took her aside to explain that Dwight seemed "speedy" and "racy," and to wonder with her if their mutual friend was "on something."

Dwight's natural shyness now became exaggerated as he withdrew inside himself, related less and less to people, and, perhaps out of embarrassment, tried to keep his medication a secret. He did not, however, increase the dose beyond the 20 mgs. each morning, a fact substantiated by his prescription records.

Although a gun collector, Dwight had not loaded and fired a gun in more than five years. Then one night about ten weeks after he started taking Prozac, he loaded a pistol, cocked it, and put it to his head. After that, he had enough presence of mind to remove the ammo from his house.

Asleep or awake, the nights became harrowing for Dwight. "They became horrible. I probably slept two or three good hours a night. I would toss and turn. When I would sleep, I had horrible, bizarre dreams of trying to crash my car, of people chasing me with knives to kill me, of confronting my ex-wife and then asking her to kill me. Many times I awoke screaming, covered with sweat, the blankets on the floor. I reached the point where I did not want to live any more. I came close to committing suicide, but in the early morning hours, I would telephone a friend, and that would calm me down."

When his prescription ran out, Dwight almost immediately became exhausted, anxious, and much more depressed. His hands would start shaking. He knew he was getting worse, but had no idea that it might be due to withdrawal. Within a week, he refilled the prescription and within three or four days felt better. In about one more month, when the prescription ran out, he again decided to go without the drug and again the symptoms returned, this time to an almost incapacitating degree. He was off medication for most of a month when he resumed taking it yet again.

Dwight's nightmares grew worse and he developed obsessive thoughts and activities. One night between 2:00 and 4:00 A.M., he went out and picked bushels of beans from his garden, illuminating the patch with his auto headlights. Although he used to hate the chore, he would iron his shirts over and over again, and sometimes get up again at night to make sure he'd done enough of them. He would also run the vacuum sweeper at all hours of the night. He remarked to me, "It's a wonder that my Hoover sweeper still has its wheels, as much and as fast as I pushed it around the house."

Dwight became so paranoid that he was afraid to enter his house at night. He heard weird whining sounds and sometimes saw the glare of lights out of the corner of his eye. He became convinced the house was occupied by evil forces, an idea that would have struck him as insanely ludicrous a few months earlier.

Although Dwight knew he was sensitive to drugs—even caffeine could make him feel wired—it did not occur to him that Prozac might be doing the same thing to him, only worse. The Prozac had helped in the beginning and he got abruptly worse when he stopped taking it. Prozac seemed like all that stood between him and insanity. Besides, when taking the drug he felt energized, and sometimes experienced feeling better and stronger than ever, as if he could do anything.

No one had warned Dwight that Prozac could cause any of the problems he was having—the agitated feelings, the insomnia and nightmares, the strange obsessive thoughts, the nausea and increasing weight loss. He would lose almost twenty pounds from his already trim frame by the time his experience with Prozac was over.

Twelve days after restarting Prozac, Dwight began the worst night of his life—leading to by far the worst day of his life and probably his ex-wife's as well. "On February

25, 1991, I slept only a few hours and once again awoke with a fearful scream from a horrible nightmare. My mind was racing. I was shaking and covered with sweat, and I felt an overpowering energy. I was so agitated, I was vomiting. I was totally out of control." He had a headache, he was shaking, and his heart was pounding. He lost track of time and the certainty of whether he was asleep or awake.

Dwight is unsure, but thinking that Prozac was his best hope, he may have taken a second pill in the early morning—at 4:00 or 5:00 A.M. He'd been vomiting most of the night and, by morning, could no longer tell if he was awake or stuck in a nightmare. "The last thing that I recall," he told me, "is that I slid down the bedroom wall and passed out on the floor." In retrospect, we know that he took two .22-caliber pistols and loaded them from a small supply of ammo he had recently found stashed away in a drawer.

Armed, Dwight went to his ex-wife's house and broke down the front door. He dragged her naked from the shower, handed her one of the guns, and begged her to shoot him. A gun went off and, although no one was hurt, it shocked Dwight into a semblance of reality. He recalled, "I saw what was going on from up above—from a corner in the ceiling of the room."

Dwight tried to reassure his terrified ex-wife that he wouldn't hurt her, and then he left the house and voluntarily admitted himself to a mental hospital.

In the hospital, Dwight's Prozac was immediately stopped, and a nurse told him it could make people "crazy" and "violent." He was tried on another antidepressant, Elavil, and a very small dose "zonked" him. He took extremely small doses for the two weeks of the hospitalization and for two weeks afterward, because they helped him sleep. He was given the very mild diagnosis of Adjustment Reaction of Adult Life—the response of an otherwise normal adult to unusual stresses. His psychological testing turned out "normal," a result I've seen in hospitalized patients only once or twice in my career.

When Dwight contacted me, he was facing five felony charges and potentially thirty-seven years in jail. In the hope of ameliorating his sentence, Dwight and his attorney decided to make a "Prozac defense" on the grounds that Prozac had contributed to his violent actions. They called upon me to give an expert opinion.

After reading his records and interviewing him for six hours, as well as interviewing people who knew him—I wrote a report to the prosecutor describing Dwight's attack on his ex-wife as a stimulant drug reaction. While there was no doubt he was angry and upset with her, and unable to let her go, I concluded that his brain had been impaired by the drug, and that he most likely would not have become violent if he had not been in a toxic, stimulant condition.

Despite the violence of Dwight's acts, his attorney, Ed Davila, was successful in making a plea bargain in which Dwight did not have to spend any time in jail. Davila believes that the Prozac defense was key. It was based on the concept of involuntary intoxication—that Dwight could not have known that the drug might influence him to commit violence and was therefore not responsible for its effect on him.

Dwight has now become the Ohio director of the Prozac Survivors Support Group, Inc. (see Appendix), and he volunteers in educating the public about Prozac. Toward that end, he gave me permission to tell his story, using his real name.

Had Dwight had better medical care—if he'd stayed in psychotherapy or been more closely monitored by his general practitioner—his toxic state might have been recognized and the medication stopped. But very likely not. Physicians have been told by Lilly and the FDA that Prozac doesn't cause severe behavioral problems like Dwight's, and many prescribing physicians don't want to believe it themselves. The truth is that many unwitting physicians might have increased Dwight's dose of Prozac when he became increasingly disturbed.

THE PARALLELS BETWEEN PROZAC AND STIMULANT DRUGS

The Basic Similarity Between Extreme Prozac and Amphetamine Responses

The story of Dwight Harlor III could have been told without changing any significant detail except for substituting amphetamine or cocaine for Prozac. Like people on speed, Dwight was initially energized in a positive fashion by Prozac, and then began to suffer insomnia and nightmares, eventually becoming isolated, paranoid, and belligerent. He began to have abnormal sensory experiences. He even became nauseated and lost weight. Dwight's clinical profile was indistinguishable from that of someone experiencing amphetamine toxicity.

It is a story I heard repeated dozens of times as I talked with Prozac survivors around the country, leading me to publish a mid-1992 Center for the Study of Psychiatry report describing the Prozac stimulant syndrome.[1] It seemed apparent that these toxic responses were largely determined by Prozac rather than by any pre-existing condition. Most of the episodes had what clinicians call an "organic flavor"—the individuals were delirious, confused, disoriented, or otherwise impaired in their brain function. In other words, the symptoms were typical of those associated with a toxic physical disorder of the brain. The reactions appeared after starting the drug, and sometimes they coincided with withdrawal.

These adverse drug reactions almost always spontaneously disappeared within weeks after drug withdrawal and without further treatment, although often there were lingering effects. If, for example, the reaction was nothing more than a manic episode unrelated to drugs, then it would rarely spontaneously improve. In addition, a number of these patients were given Prozac not for depression but for other problems, including fatigue, weight loss, and obsessions and compulsions.

Some individuals also became suicidal and violent while on Prozac without having the full-blown stimulant syndrome that I have described. I have seen this in my own practice. This, too, can be found in amphetamine reactions.

The major adverse effects of the amphetamines—like those of Prozac—are exaggerations of the desired effects, specifically stimulation, including insomnia, anxiety, and hyperactivity. The most common drawback to continuing amphetamine from the user's perspective is the activation syndrome—"the hand-wringing, pacing, and excess energy may produce an acute anxiety reaction."[2] As is now commonly done with Prozac, amphetamines were often prescribed along with a sedative to relieve overstimulation.

Had the FDA followed the conclusions of the March 1986 "Safety Review" by its own expert, Richard Kapit (see page 74), and required a warning about Prozac's stimulant effects, tragedies like Dwight's would be much less likely to occur. Most physicians know that stimulants like the amphetamines and cocaine can produce agitation, paranoia, and violence, and they would have been alerted to the same dangerous possibility with Prozac.

It will be helpful to review the capacity of both the classic stimulants and the SSRIs to produce abnormal behavior such as paranoia, violence, depression, and suicide. The comparison to stimulants confirms that drugs can indeed produce these dangerous behavioral effects, and helps us to anticipate the dangerous effects of the SSRIs before they become fully documented. It also underscores that the drug companies, the FDA, and the psychiatric profession tend to resist recognizing the dangerous behavioral effects from psychoactive prescription drugs.

While nonpsychiatric physicians are also responsible for this problem, they tend to follow the lead of psychiatric experts.

Stimulants and Prozac Both Cause Compulsive Behavior

We have seen how Prozac users can develop bizarre compulsions. They may spend hours cleaning windows from the outside in the dark or simply cleaning house. Many speed users also develop compulsive and seemingly meaningless repetitive activities, such as polishing and fondling stones or beads for hours on end, or taking machinery apart and putting it back together again. Sometimes "speeders" devote days to activities like polishing a car or making drawings full of minutia. Sometimes the compulsive activities become self-destructive, as in skin-picking.[3]

The compulsiveness in part reflects a drug-induced narrowing of focus[4] that may be related to stereotypical behavior in animals produced by the same drugs. Stereotypical behavior in animals involves purposeless, repetitive voluntary movements that are carried out for periods of time at the expense of all other activities. Rats may spend inordinate amounts of time licking, gnawing, or sniffing, while dogs or chimpanzees may compulsively run or walk around in a repetitive fashion.[5]

This stereotypical behavior, with its compulsive attention to very limited or boring tasks, may be the sought-after effect in giving amphetamines, including Ritalin, to schoolchildren. Compulsiveness also is an aspect of Prozac-induced violence and suicide.

Stimulants and Prozac Both Cause Violence

In 1980 the National Institute of Drug Abuse (NIDA) published a compendium of reports on *Use and Abuse of Amphetamine and Its Substitutes,* edited by James and Carol Spotts. The editors point out: "Initially it was thought that there were no serious adverse psychological effects associated with the use of therapeutic doses of amphetamine."[6] However, they remark, as early as 1938, cases of paranoid psychosis were reported in routine medical use. The problem came to a head over the use of relatively low-dose Benzedrine inhalers for respiratory problems. While predisposing factors may play a role, Spotts and Spotts emphasize that minimal doses (5 to 10 mgs. of amphetamine)[7] can cause psychosis—an important consideration in evaluating reports of abnormal reactions on relatively low doses of Prozac.

Spotts and Spotts put it succinctly: "Reports of incidents of violence and aggression by amphetamine abusers permeate the research literature."[8] Roger Smith from the Department of Pharmacology at the University of California stated the following at a 1970 conference on amphetamines sponsored by the National Institute of Mental Health (NIMH): "[T]he literature is replete with accounts of violent behavior by individuals using oral amphetamines in isolation."

During the 1954 to 1956 Japanese epidemic of amphetamine use, more than 50 percent of sixty murders occurring in Japan in a two-month period were connected with amphetamine abuse. The slogan "Speed Kills" referred in part to the murderousness sometimes induced by the drug.

Amphetamine expert E. H. Ellinwood, Jr., M.D., from the Duke University Department of Psychiatry, "observed several cases in which amphetamine-induced paranoid delusional thinking, panic, emotional lability, or lowered impulse control was directly related to the series of events leading to a homicide."[9] Some of the main characteristics of people taking amphetamine included "suspiciousness, hyperactivity, and lability [instability] of mood." They become "suspicious of their family, friends, strangers, and lovers." John Kramer, M.D., from the Orange County Medical Center in California, concluded that there can be little or no doubt that these stimulants produce violence where it might not otherwise occur. Amphetamine withdrawal can also precipitate increased paranoia and violence.[10]

Although the American Psychiatric Association tends to be very supportive of pharmaceuticals, its 1987 diagnostic manual, the *DSM-III-R,* confirms the danger of violence associated with stimulant drugs, such as Dexedrine and Ritalin.[11]

Stimulants and Prozac Both Can Cause Depression and Suicide

As early as 1966, the American Medical Association issued a formal warning about amphetamine dependence, noting that withdrawal can "trigger a depressive or schizophrenic reaction, sometimes with suicidal potential." A recent chapter on the abuse of stimulants in *Treatments of Psychiatric Disorders* (1989) reconfirms, "The depression of the crash can be extremely intense and may include potentially lethal, but temporary, suicidal ideation [thinking], which remits completely when the crash is over."[12] Notice that the suicidality is drug-induced and disappears when the drug wears off.

Pallie Carnes: A Close Call on Prozac

Pallie Carnes is an example of a patient who might have been saved from tragedy had her physician been aware of the Prozac stimulant syndrome. She testified at the 1991 FDA Prozac hearing about how she had been prescribed Prozac for weight loss.

In a personal interview this year with Ginger Breggin, Pallie reported that she had no previous psychiatric history prior to starting Prozac. Her doctor prescribed the drug as a diet pill because she was sixteen pounds overweight, and never told her it was an antidepressant psychiatric drug.

At the FDA hearings, she testified:

> I was put on Prozac for weight loss, since I had had a baby the year before and I was having a hard time getting the stubborn pounds off. . . . [A]nd only three days after being put on Prozac I started having terrifying nightmares. I would wake up screaming and the nightmares always had something to do with death.
>
> I couldn't laugh and I couldn't cry. I started having headaches and forgetfulness. I had no emotions at all. Soon after, I started having suicidal thoughts, followed by a suicide attempt. I was always very agitated with the people I had to deal with on a daily basis. My friends and family were very concerned about me. My children did not understand what was happening to their mother. I didn't realize what I was putting them through. And to top it all off, I gained weight.
>
> Then, from watching a TV talk show, I learned that Prozac was an antidepressant drug and not a weight-loss aid and that a lot of people taking Prozac were having the same symptoms that I was having. I quit taking Prozac that day, and soon after, I started feeling like my own self again. . . .
>
> I was a different person while I was taking Prozac. I was a zombie. I would sit and stare. I was completely without emotions. If you can only realize how this feels, not to be able to laugh or cry and not know why. I didn't have the patience to help my children with their homework or the energy to play a game with them like I usually do. But I didn't care. I only knew that I did not want to be around anyone, and that included my family. . . .

Eli Lilly calls Prozac the wonder drug, and I wonder why. Thinking back on how this drug affected me, does a wonder drug rob you of a conscience? Does a wonder drug make you forget the difference between right and wrong? I no longer wonder about this so-called wonder drug; I now know that I wouldn't be here today if I continued taking this killer drug. . . .

I tried to commit suicide in front of my five children. I didn't know what I was doing and don't remember exactly what happened. All I know is that my husband took the gun away from me and my children were looking in from the other room.

What would have happened if these children had seen their mother commit suicide? I was only put on it for weight loss—weight loss. Is it worth it for my children to be motherless today because of a drug that has no side effects, I was told—had no side effects—but yet it brought me to the brink of holding a gun to my head and almost killing myself.

Although Pallie was unaware of the significance of it until we questioned her, she had undergone Prozac-induced stimulant side effects, including violent nightmares, sleeplessness, and lack of concentration. She felt "shaky inside, like panicky," but outside she was a "zombie." She felt "speeded up on the inside, but not on the outside," except for pacing a great deal. At times she was obsessed with suicide. For the first and only time in her life, she found herself compulsively washing and rewashing her hands.

Once Pallie stopped taking Prozac, her symptoms immediately began to clear up, although the fatigue, headaches, and forgetfulness lasted for some time. She feels her life has finally returned to normal.

Stimulants and Prozac Both Are Reuptake Blockers

From early on, it was apparent that three neurotransmitter systems are potentially involved in amphetamine-induced behavioral and mental abnormalities—dopamine, norepinephrine, and serotonin—all of which are energized by amphetamines and cocaine.[13] Cocaine is known to block the reuptake* of dopamine, norepinephrine, and serotonin in the brain, amplifying the impact of these neurotransmitter systems. Amphetamines also block the reuptake of these three neurotransmitters, more especially dopamine. Prozac more specifically blocks the reuptake of serotonin, but also affects dopamine and norepinephrine.

Patients sometimes report hallucinogenic experiences while taking SSRIs, amphetamines, and other drugs that stimulate serotonin nerves.[14]

In 1986, researcher Kurt Rasmussen and his colleagues at the Yale University School of Medicine found that the power of many hallucinogenic drugs was proportional to their activity at serotonergic receptors. In his book *Food of the Gods,* Terence McKenna points out that many hallucinogenic substances, such as LSD and hallucinogenic mushrooms, are chemically related to serotonin and its precursor tryptophan.[15] Psychologist Donald Templer and his co-authors observed in 1992 that "it is generally believed that the hallucinogenic properties of many other drugs (such as MDMA, mescaline, and psilocybin) are due to their interaction with serotonin systems in the brain."

A SUMMARY OF THE SIMILARITIES BETWEEN STIMULANTS AND PROZAC

A point-by-point summary of the comparisons between the classical stimulants and Prozac presents ominous parallels.

*Reuptake is described in chapter 2.

- Both groups of drugs produce stimulant syndromes in routine use.
- Both were quickly and widely embraced with testimonials by doctors and patients concerning near-miraculous mood-elevating effects.
- Both continue to be prescribed by many physicians who claim that patients experience few side effects and no withdrawal problems.
- Both reached epidemic proportions of prescription use.
- Both can produce very dangerous behavioral aberrations.
- Both are reuptake blockers that cause abnormal hyperactivity of serotonergic nerves and impact as well on the dopaminergic and adrenergic nerves.
- Both have repeatedly been whitewashed by their respective drug companies and the FDA.

The history of the pharmaceutical industry and the FDA in regard to amphetamines is telling. Physicians and much of the public know that stimulants are very dangerous drugs, yet the pharmaceutical industry and the FDA have been slow to mandate public warnings. The evidence is mounting regarding the potential of Prozac to cause many of the same devastating side effects—including violence and suicide—of the stimulants. One wonders how long it will take for the FDA or Eli Lilly to provide adequate warnings regarding Prozac.

Finally, don't forget that the Appendix provides you or your doctor with the form for reporting an adverse drug reaction directly to the FDA.

SEVEN

Can Prozac Cause Violence and Suicide?

What Survivors, Independent Researchers, and the FDA Have to Say

On September 20, 1991, the FDA held a hearing to determine whether or not antidepressants in general can cause destructive behavioral reactions such as suicide and murder.[1] The hearings were called because of the enormous media attention generated by a combination of spectacular murders committed by persons taking Prozac and by a Harvard research team's clinical report describing six cases of Prozac-induced compulsive, violently suicidal thoughts.

BACKGROUND OF THE HEARINGS

The manufacturers of each of the many antidepressants were invited to make presentations at the September 1991 Prozac hearing, but Eli Lilly was the only one to respond. At issue was whether or not the drug company should be required to change the Prozac label to include a warning that the drug could cause or worsen violence against self or others.

The final determination regarding Prozac's label would be made by the FDA, in particular, by psychiatrist Paul Leber, longtime director of the FDA's Division of Neuropharmacological Drug Products. The hearing was held before the FDA's advisory committee on psychopharmaceuticals, a group of experts that the FDA itself selects. A number of FDA-chosen consultants were also invited.

The hearing began with public testimony, some of which has been included as case history throughout this book. Various interested organizations also gave testimony, most of them representing organized psychiatry. They warned against creating public doubt about the safety and efficacy of psychiatric drugs. FDA representatives and a series of experts brought in by Eli Lilly also testified.

The one-day hearing concluded with the nine-member FDA committee voting unanimously that there was no "credible evidence" that antidepressants can induce or intensify violence and suicide. Then, with one-third of its members dissenting, the committee made a divided decision *against* any label change drawing greater attention to the problem.

Following the hearing, the public was told that the subject had been laid to rest: Prozac and the other SSRIs, including Zoloft and Paxil, do not cause violence or suicide. But the public was *not* told about the amount of controversy or the conflicts of interest among many of the professionals gathered at the hearing.* Nor was the public informed of the nature and extent of independent research findings, as well as the nightmarish personal experiences of Prozac users, that led to the FDA hearings.

THE WESBECKER MASS-MURDER CASE

The story of Joseph Wesbecker caught the nation's attention and helped to bring about the FDA hearing.† Ac-

---

*The conflicts of interest represented by many of the FDA-selected committee members will be documented in chapter 8.

†Because of my role as a medical expert for the plaintiffs in product-

cording to the November 1990 issue of the *ABA Journal*, published by the American Bar Association:[2]

> Before Joseph Wesbecker burst into a Louisville, Kentucky, printing plant in September 1989 with an AK-47 assault rifle, he had taken an antidepressant called Prozac, touted in some press reports as a wonder drug with few side effects. After killing eight people and wounding 12 others, he turned the gun on himself.

The victims who survived the shooting, relatives of the deceased, and Wesbecker's own family began to bring suits against Eli Lilly, claiming that "Prozac, one of the drug manufacturer's biggest moneymakers, is partly responsible for the gunman's violent actions." The suits, according to the *ABA Journal*, "allege that Eli Lilly knew or should have known that Prozac was unsafe for use by the general public for the treatment of depression. They also charged the company knew or should have known that users of the drug can experience intense agitation and preoccupation with suicide, and can harm themselves or others."

Wesbecker had been prescribed Prozac on August 3, 1989. Five weeks later, Wesbecker's Louisville psychiatrist, Lee Coleman, noticed a dramatic change for the worse in his patient during a routine visit. Confirming a now-familiar theme, Coleman testified at the inquest[3] that Wesbecker was "very, very agitated" at his last session. Coleman described him as "much more nervous and anxious than he normally was." He was also having increased sleep problems. Speaking specifically of Prozac, Coleman further testified, "Some of the nervousness and anxiety, I

---

liability suits against Eli Lilly related to Wesbecker's actions, I cannot become involved in a lengthy discussion of the case. Nor can this brief summary provide the reader adequate detail to make an informed decision about the merits of any of the cases. I have cited only documents that are available to the public. The case is currently scheduled to come to trial in September 1994 but may be postponed.

felt, were probably side effects of his medication." Thinking that Prozac could be the cause of the agitation, Coleman told Wesbecker to stop taking it.

Wesbecker himself thought Prozac was helping. But Coleman testified, "because of his deterioration, he needed to stop that medication."

In his office notes on Wesbecker's last visit, Coleman wrote that Wesbecker was suffering from an "increased level of agitation and anger" and indicated that he suspected Prozac was the cause. He urged hospitalization but Wesbecker refused. Three days later, on September 14, 1989, still with a high level of Prozac in his blood, Wesbecker carried a gun into his former workplace and committed mayhem.

Wesbecker had a past history of psychiatric hospitalizations, threats of violence, and suicide attempts. He was taking other psychiatric drugs along with the Prozac and had a therapeutic level of lithium in his system. He had been prescribed Prozac once before in the summer of 1988 but had quit taking it after less than three weeks because of fatigue.

Coleman testified that he did not believe Wesbecker's violence could be attributed to Prozac. He considered Prozac "an excellent drug" and he was continuing to prescribe the medication to increasing numbers of patients.

A friend of Wesbecker's, James Robert Lukas, Sr., testified at the inquest that he had known Wesbecker for twenty-nine years. Lukas himself had become impulsively violent while taking Prozac. After seven weeks of treatment, he tried to stab his wife with a ballpoint pen. While on the drug, he did not perceive his own irrationality; but after the attempted stabbing, Lukas's wife called his psychiatrist, who immediately took Lukas off Prozac.

Lukas became concerned and then frightened when he saw Wesbecker's personality transformed while taking Prozac. His old friend became a different person and was so threatening that Lukas called people at work to warn them of the danger.

Lilly has denied the charges made in the various Wesbecker suits. The company told the *ABA Journal*: "Our experience does not show a cause and effect relationship between our products and suicidal or violent thoughts or acts. Unfortunately, these thoughts and acts are part of the disease of depression." Eli Lilly did revise its Prozac package insert in May 1990 and then the 1991 *Physicians' Desk Reference* to warn that "suicidal ideation" and "violent behavior" had been reported by some who took the drug. Lilly did not, however, confirm a *causal* relationship between the drug and these behaviors.

The Wesbecker case and the publicity around it was one of the critical factors in prompting the FDA to hold hearings in the fall of 1991.

THE FLOODGATE OF PROZAC HORROR STORIES

The two years leading up to and overlapping the FDA hearing, 1990–1, saw an enormous amount of media and legal attention focused on Prozac. As Prozac horror stories flooded the media, an increasing number of lawsuits (a total of 170 by the end of 1992) were filed against Eli Lilly. Others exposed to Prozac argued in court that their violent actions had been fueled by Prozac. In some cases, at least, this "Prozac defense" seemed to result in lighter sentences.[4]

Among the events reported in 1990 are the following:

- In 1990 the Prozac Survivors Support Group asked the Bucks County, Pennsylvania, coroner to reopen the investigation into political activist Abbie Hoffman's suicide to see if he was driven to it by Prozac.[5]
- The *New York Times* reported that El Sayyid A. Nosair was taking Prozac for depression at the time he

allegedly murdered Rabbi Meir Kahane, the controversial founder of the Jewish Defense League.*[6]

- A woman reported withdrawing into herself while on Prozac and plotting the death of her four children, while another woman on Prozac acted on her feelings and killed a friend and then herself.[7]
- Another woman sued Eli Lilly on the grounds that Prozac, given to her as a pick-me-up, made her suicidal and homicidal.[8]
- A woman who held her psychiatrist "hostage" with a razor to her own wrist sued Lilly concerning self-mutilations inflicted while taking Prozac.[9]
- A defense attorney argued that a former teacher, while under the influence of Prozac, shot a woman to death.[10]
- Joe and Teresa Graedon reported on August 10, 1990, in their syndicated column, "The People's Pharmacy," that they had received "15 reports of individuals who attempted or committed suicide while they were taking Prozac."

Reports linking Prozac to violence flooded the media during 1991, the year of the FDA hearing. In this section, we review those that were brought to our attention, mostly through the efforts of Dwight Harlor III and other Prozac survivors, who collected the clippings.

Violence perpetrated while taking Prozac was the most common theme:†

- A judge sentenced a man who killed his father to only four years' probation on the grounds that the father had been driven into a frenzy by Prozac.[11]

---

*He was acquitted of murder.
†In some of these cases we were not able to ascertain if the individuals were ultimately found innocent and therefore the newspaper clippings we cite do not establish whether or not they committed the alleged conduct.

- An elementary-school teacher, while taking Prozac for depression, stabbed his estranged wife.[12]
- A seventy-six-year-old woman who became "increasingly irritable, anxiety-ridden and delusional during the 3½ weeks she took Prozac" was convicted of shooting her husband while he slept, but received probation despite the prosecution's demand for a jail sentence.[13]
- A fifty-year-old man with no violence in his background became distraught over his divorce, was put on Prozac, and one week later shot his ex-wife's boyfriend in the chest.[14]
- A thirty-nine-year-old woman suffered a striking personality change on Prozac, including "distraction, extreme agitation, restlessness, insomnia, homicidal ideation and actions," and strangled her mother to death.[15]
- A man who strangled his girlfriend made a Prozac defense.[16]
- A woman accused of deliberately running down and killing a child with her car pleaded that Prozac was the cause.[17]
- During a domestic quarrel a man on Prozac shot and killed his wife.[18]
- A woman on Prozac axed her husband to death, set him on fire, and then shot herself in the head with a hunting rifle.[19]
- A sixty-one-year-old woman, a university professor, took bone-deep bites out of her elderly mother, declaring "she made me mad, so mad, I've been taking Prozac for the last two weeks."[20]
- A man accused of killing his estranged wife and her male friend recently had had his Prozac dose doubled, changing his behavior, according to witnesses.[21]
- A man on Prozac broke into the house of another man, who was dating his ex-wife, and beat him with a flashlight; he received only a misdemeanor conviction from the jury.[22]
- A mother who shot her two sons and her husband to

death attributed it to her taking Prozac for twenty-one days.[23]

- A woman responsible for a fatal auto accident was given a light sentence, the judge explained, because she was taking Prozac at the time.[24]
- A woman facing felony charges in the hit-and-run death of a cyclist was on Prozac.[25]
- A man, after missing his daily dose of Prozac and drinking heavily, shot a thirteen-year-old girl in the arm.[26]
- "High on a combination of crack cocaine and the antidepressant drug Prozac," a man stabbed his wife and then attacked a policeman head on, forcing the officer to shoot him to death.[27]
- A self-described "manic depressive" and disgruntled employee had been off Prozac for one week when he set a revenge fire that injured twenty-one people.[28]
- A woman testified about her grandson—"He was a different person when he used Prozac. He was shaky. He got angry quickly"—in explanation for why he tried to strangle his wife and later threatened suicide.[29]
- A Canadian taking Prozac ran his car at another man and fired his gun into the air following an altercation at a gas station; a psychiatrist testified that Prozac caused the hypomanic behavior.[30]
- A man on Prozac allegedly hired someone to kill his wife.[31]
- When a man became increasingly irritable on Prozac, his psychiatrist doubled the dose, and the man stabbed his wife in the throat and back with a kitchen knife.[32]
- A woman shot the doctor who was giving her Prozac, but she liked him and couldn't explain why she had done it.[33]

Many of the 1991 media stories involved suicide, sometimes in combination with violence against others:

- Former rock star Del Shannon committed suicide in Los Angeles while taking Prozac; his wife brought suit against Eli Lilly.[34]
- A mother reported that her daughter had burned herself to death while taking Prozac.[35]
- A twenty-year-old man taking Prozac for depression jumped off a ten-story parking garage.[36]
- An attorney brought suit against Eli Lilly for the suicide of his wife, who had been taking Prozac at the time.[37]
- A woman brought suit against the drug manufacturer for the "incomprehensible" suicide of her husband during treatment with Prozac.[38]
- A fifteen-year-old Eagle Scout was taking Prozac when he shot himself in the head with a shotgun.[39]
- A woman sued Lilly, attributing her suicide attempt to Prozac.[40]
- A twenty-nine-year-old mother of two taking Prozac set the table for dinner and started making gravy, but when her husband arrived home, he found her hanging by a belt in the bedroom.[41]
- A depressed woman became hostile while taking Prozac the first time and, when placed on it again, committed suicide.[42]

As illustrated by yet more 1991 media reports, sometimes the violence against others ended in suicide:

- A former sheriff's deputy murdered his wife and then shot himself while on Prozac.[43]
- A thirty-year-old woman being treated with Prozac for depression shot her baby in the head several times and then killed herself.[44]
- Two days after stopping his Prozac, a pathologist who suffered from alcoholism shot his wife and then killed himself with a razor.[45]

Other 1991 media-reported stories showed an increasing tendency to use the Prozac defense for crime and violence:

- A librarian accused of making irregular expenditures claimed that Prozac impaired her judgment so that she "didn't know the boundary between herself and the library."[46]
- A desperate woman awaiting her first welfare check was taking Prozac when she robbed a bank without a weapon. She was easily caught and received probation.[47]
- A man armed with an air pistol robbed a store and blamed his behavior on Prozac, while another man in the same court refused to use the Prozac defense in regard to his fraudulent activities.[48]
- A woman claimed she became a nymphomaniac and turned to prostitution while taking Prozac.[49]

On April 22, 1991, five months before the FDA Prozac hearing, syndicated health columnists Joe and Teresa Graedon cited one of their earlier columns and reported that: "Since then we have received dozens of letters from people who believe Prozac in some way contributed to severe anxiety, violent behavior or a preoccupation with suicide. Eli Lilly, the drug company, steadfastly maintains that Prozac is not responsible. But we are concerned."

The media usually provides too few details to develop an informed opinion about the role played by Prozac in any particular case. What's striking is the sheer number of reports associating the drug with violence against self and others. While other medications, especially amphetamines and minor tranquilizers such as Halcion, have been linked to destructive behavior, there's no precedent for this avalanche of media reports pertaining to a prescription drug.

FAMILY TESTIMONY AT THE
FDA PROZAC HEARING

Tragic Prozac stories were told in more elaborate—and heartrending—detail at the FDA Prozac hearing in September 1991. Here are three examples from family members.

Mrs. Margaret McCaffrey traveled from Brooklyn, New York, to testify:

> I raised eight children. Two of them became doctors. My daughter, Margaret, a neurologist, died a little over a year ago and I firmly believe the drug Prozac caused her to commit suicide. She was very dedicated to her profession. She was a nurse before going to medical school. She took Prozac to see her through a very stressful job situation. . . .
>
> She moved to Baltimore in July of 1990 to begin a second fellowship. She had bought a new car, had a lovely apartment, and the best of her profession lay ahead. There was no warning. She spoke to her family on Saturday and on Monday morning she was found, almost dead.
>
> I hope and pray that Eli Lilly and the FDA will listen to me and remove this drug from the market before any more innocent lives are lost. Thank you.

When Ginger Breggin contacted Mrs. McCaffrey, she was grateful that we were looking into the Prozac matter, and said that her daughter's fiancé has filed suit against Eli Lilly.

D.M.* explained that her father had been taking Prozac for about four months when tragedy struck:

> Unfortunately, with my dad we didn't have time to notice too many changes, except that he became withdrawn and

---

*While the story is in the public domain, we have not been able to talk directly to D.M. or her father, and so we are, in this case, using made-up initials.

agitated. But by that time it was too late. He got up at 9 o'clock in the morning, took a 12-inch butcher knife out of the kitchen drawer and stabbed himself violently in the abdomen and then proceeded to do it twice more.

D.M.'s father was caught in the act and his life was saved, but he had to undergo months of painful recovery.[50]

The widow of pop singer Del Shannon also testified. Unlike most of the others who spoke at the hearing, she displayed a rather sophisticated knowledge about the drug and its effects. The musician's reaction to Prozac was very similar to that of Dwight Harlor III:

Before Prozac, my husband was very involved with people, our family, and his work. He was very much in charge of his business. But within days after he started taking Prozac I noticed a personality change in him. He showed signs of restlessness, akathisia,* agitation, pacing, and his appearance was very drawn. He developed severe insomnia, extreme fatigue, chills, racing heart, dry mouth, and upset stomach. His hands would shake uncontrollably at times. This really alarmed him. I would ask him what was wrong and his only reply was, "I don't know."

Like many cases drawn to my attention, Del Shannon's act seemed inexplicably impulsive. He left no suicide note and he had appointments and gigs lined up for the coming days. He asked the family to pick up some vitamins for him on their way to the market, and then shot himself dead before they got back. He had been on Prozac for fifteen days.

As the last two stories reconfirm, Prozac-induced violence and suicide are often associated with feelings of agitation. Frequently the person seems "jittery," "hyper," "driven," anxious, and withdrawn.

---

*Discussed in chapter 4 and later in this chapter.

PROZAC SURVIVORS: THE OFFICIAL TALLY

At my request, Bonnie Leitsch, then director of the national Prozac Survivors Support Group, summarized all the reports coming into the organization during 1991 and 1992. The information covered 288 individuals who had adverse reactions to Prozac during those two years.*

The vast majority were related to violence against self or others. There were 164 cases in the suicide and suicide ideation category, including 34 completed suicides. There were 133 cases of crime and violence, including 14 murders (6 by gun, 5 by car), 9 attempted murders, 39 violent actions (8 in cars), 54 violent preoccupations (5 in cars), and 17 crimes.

There were 13 reports of addiction to Prozac and 14 cases of alcohol abuse developing or worsening on Prozac.

Bonnie was impressed, as I have been, by the number of references to experiences associated with automobiles. Perhaps agitation and hyperactivity are especially susceptible to aggravation within the confines of a car and under the stresses of driving.

In reviewing the media and survivor group reports on violence, and in the literature that we shall now examine, keep in mind that violence and murder are quite rare among depressed patients.[51] It is not possible to attribute so much violence to depression itself.

RESEARCH DISCOVERIES ABOUT PROZAC FOLLOWING ITS APPROVAL BY THE FDA

During this same time period surrounding the FDA hearings, a variety of pharmaceutical and medical sources be-

*As of March 1994, she had logged over 1,000 cases.

gan to acknowledge suicide and/or violence as potential problems from Prozac.[52]

The Teicher, Glod, and Cole Report

The outpouring of media reports of Prozac-induced murder and suicide gained confirmation from a publication in the February 1990 *American Journal of Psychiatry*, and this inspired a wave of further reports and controversy in the medical literature. Written by two well-known Harvard psychiatrists, Martin Teicher and Jonathan Cole, and a nurse, Carol Glod, the clinical report described six Prozac-treated patients[53] who developed "intense, violent suicidal preoccupations" within two to seven weeks of starting treatment with Prozac. "None of these patients had ever experienced a similar state during treatment with any other psychotropic drug." The feelings seemed obsessive and emerged without apparent reason or provocation. One of the patients actually put a loaded gun to her head and another needed physical restraint to prevent self-mutilation.

Based on their clinical experience, Teicher, Glod, and Cole estimated that between 1.9 and 7.7 percent of Prozac users would be afflicted with obsessive or violent suicidal thoughts. The article gained importance not only because of the stature of the two psychiatrists, Teicher and Cole, but also because Cole himself had been a clinical investigator for Eli Lilly in clinical trials of Prozac.

Teicher's report quickly met resistance and even anger from within the profession. Richard Miller, a Hartford, Connecticut, psychiatrist, pointed out that four of Teicher's six patients were taking other drugs, including two who were on stimulants.[54] Miller concluded, "Fluoxetine is a revolutionary antidepressant with many effective uses. Its relative lack of side effects is impressive."

Without identifying himself as an employee of Eli Lilly, in a letter to the *American Journal of Psychiatry*, psychiatrist Gary Tollefson expressed fear that the Teicher article "may introduce a medical-legal precedent." In their rebuttal, Teicher, Glod, and Cole took Tollefson to task for placing self-protective medical-legal concerns ahead of patient care, research, and teaching. Admitting their evidence was not "definitive," the Harvard group stood by their report.

In response to Teicher's article, Harvard psychiatrists Maurizio Fava and Jerrold Rosenbaum used questionnaires to survey twenty-seven psychiatrists associated with the Massachusetts General Hospital. The doctors had treated 1,017 depressed patients. A total of twelve patients were described as having become suicidal after starting medication—six of them on fluoxetine. Fava and Rosenbaum reported that the higher rate on Prozac was not statistically significant.[55]

Teicher, Glod, and Cole reviewed Fava and Rosenbaum's data and found fault with their statistical analysis.[56] Prozac patients were, in fact, "at least three-fold more likely to develop new suicidal ideation" than patients treated with the older antidepressants. Patients were also more likely to develop suicidal thoughts *for the first time ever* while taking Prozac.

At the FDA hearings, Teicher reviewed an older study demonstrating a very large increase in suicide on tricyclic antidepressants.[57] He then briefly explained the actual results of the Fava and Rosenbaum study to the agency's psychopharmacology committee. But when he tried to show some slides to prove his point, committee chairman Daniel Casey, a Portland psychiatrist and professor at the University of Oregon, refused to allow him to do so.[58] Instead, chairman Casey interrupted to announce his own opinion that there was no evidence that antidepressants could cause the emergence or intensification of suicidal or violent behaviors, and then he called for a committee vote.

Paul Leber, Director of the Division of Neuropharmacological Drug Products of the FDA, had already stated that there was insufficient evidence to conclude that Prozac was causing behavioral aberrations. He did this immediately following the heartrending testimonials and before the panel of handpicked FDA experts had heard any professional testimony or begun its deliberation.[59]

Teicher never got to show his slides.

Teicher, however, was not alone in the profession.

In testimony given on behalf of a defendant in a murder trial on November 15, 1990, Teicher stated that he had received a great number of additional calls and letters from patients, families, and physicians confirming his report on Prozac-induced suicidality.[60]

In *Drug Safety* in 1993, Teicher's group reconfirmed the increasing number of reports they were receiving and published a comprehensive review of ways in which Prozac can cause suicide or violence. They presented yet another case, this time a woman who became obsessed with murdering members of her family.

In a letter in December 1990, Teicher and his colleagues reported that they had received communications from two psychiatrists describing "the emergence of suicidal ideation that began two weeks after initiation of fluoxetine (20 mg) to treat obsessive features in three adolescents with Tourette's disorder." Another physician sent them a report of "suicide by hanging that occurred two weeks after initiation of fluoxetine (20 mg) in a fifteen-year-old adolescent with obsessive-compulsive disorder who had little or no preexisting depression."[61]

By the time the hearings were held in the fall of 1991, there was already a great deal of confirmatory evidence to support the Harvard group's original observations. And at the hearing, Teicher reported that he had data on two patients whose mental condition once again deteriorated on rechallenge (restarting of the drug) and that he was aware of eight such cases.[62]

Teicher's report, meanwhile, may have had some impact on Eli Lilly and the FDA because, on May 29, 1990, "suicidal ideation" and "violent behaviors" were added to the official Prozac label under "Postintroduction Reports." Appearing for the first time in the *Physicians' Desk Reference* in 1991, the section begins with a caveat that no "causal relationship" had been proven between the drug and the specific behavioral reactions. The hearing focused on whether or not Prozac *caused* violence and suicide.

The Public Citizen Health Research Group, a Ralph Nader–affiliated organization, is directed by physician Sidney Wolfe. In May 1991, and based largely on Teicher's findings, the group petitioned the FDA to add a warning to Prozac's label stating that "A small minority of persons taking fluoxetine have experienced intense, violent, suicidal thoughts, agitation, and impulsivity after starting treatment with the drug."[63] The petition was eventually rejected by the FDA.

The Unpublished Geller Data

In a follow-up letter published in the November 1990 issue of the *American Journal of Psychiatry*, Teicher and his Harvard team made another startling disclosure: that a Prozac trial of depressed adolescents conducted by psychiatrist Barbara Geller at the University of South Carolina had to be abruptly terminated because of the "emergence of intense violent suicidal and/or homicidal ideation in five patients."[*64]

---

*A September 1991 letter to the *American Journal of Psychiatry* by Harriet Fetner, Pharm.D.; Hazel E. Watts, B.S.N.; and Barbara Geller, M.D., from Columbia, South Carolina, corrected Teicher's characterization of Geller's remarks to him. They reported they had not conducted any formal "protocol" or "investigation" but that they did have "routine clinical experience with fluoxetine." Oddly, their letter neither confirms nor denies Teicher's statement that Geller shared with him several clinical experiences with youngsters who became suicidal or violent on Prozac. Despite the ambiguities of their letter, the three authors hope that Teicher's error will not "in any way alter" the importance of his work.

More Medical Reports on the Dark Side of Prozac

Anecdotal reports confirming Teicher, Glod, and Cole began to appear in 1990 and 1991.[65] Psychiatrist Prakash Masand and colleagues in Syracuse, New York, reported in the *New England Journal of Medicine* on two cases of suicidality that seemed clearly related to Prozac. Later, in defense of Prozac, Masand called it a "very real but small risk."[66] New York psychiatrists Laszlo Papp and Jack Gorman described a paradoxical transient worsening of their patients' obsessions and compulsions early in Prozac treatment, and suspected that this reaction contributed to the suicidality of some of Teicher's patients.[67]

In July 1991, Hisako Koizumi, M.D., from the Harding Hospital in Worthington, Ohio, reported in the *Journal of Child and Adolescent Psychiatry* on the case of a thirteen-year-old boy who became "full of energy," "hyperactive," and "clown-like" in behavior while taking Prozac. On doses below the recommended level he developed violent, explosive behavior that was "totally unlike him."

Again in 1991, C. Thomas Gualtieri, an experienced research psychiatrist from Chapel Hill, North Carolina, "reviewed the case of a mentally handicapped gentleman whose rates of self-injurious behavior doubled on fluoxetine, and then fell to baseline after the drug was withdrawn." Noting the enormous complexity of Prozac's effects on the brain, Gualtieri observed that Prozac's effects can run the spectrum from "apathy" to "mania." He concluded, "Unpredictable responses may well be a predictable characteristic of drugs like fluoxetine. . . ."

In 1991, a psychiatric group led by W. Creaney from the Academic Unit of the North Wales Hospital described two cases of suicidal reactions attributed to Prozac and to fluvoxamine, a European SSRI. One patient eventually became, in his own words, "helpless, ill, mentally restless, beyond repair and suicidal." The second patient became more actively suicidal, and both initially failed to realize that the medication was making them worse.

Timothy Brewerton at the Medical University of South Carolina reviewed studies indicating suicidality and depression caused by Prozac and concluded that rapid changes in serotonin concentration are probably the cause.

Other reports on mania due to Prozac were overlooked in the controversy because hostility or violence was not their main theme.[68] Still other reports confirmed that patients can become paranoid on Prozac.[69]

The Yale Reports on Children and Adolescents

As the controversy over Prozac and suicide heated up, Robert A. King and a team from the Yale University School of Medicine published a March 1991 report on the "Emergence of Self-Destructive Phenomena in Children and Adolescents During Fluoxetine Treatment." Because young people were involved, the cases were less complicated than Teicher's. "Self-injurious ideation or behavior appeared de novo [for the first time] or intensified" in six of forty-seven patients being treated with Prozac for obsessive-compulsive disorder. Four of the cases required hospitalization and three required "restraints, seclusion, or one-to-one nursing care."

In a second study, published in the 1990–1 issue of the *Journal of Child and Adolescent Psychopharmacology*, psychiatrist Mark Riddle and the same Yale group found that twelve of twenty-four children and adolescents, ages eight to sixteen, developed two or more behavioral side effects in reaction to Prozac. Most of the youngsters were being treated for obsessive-compulsive symptoms. The drug-induced effects included motor restlessness sufficient to cause concern to parents or teachers, insomnia, social disinhibition manifested by garrulousness or subtle impulsivity, and a subjective sense of discomfort due to restlessness, agitation, or excessive energy. The group included three children with attention deficit hyperactivity disorder (ADHD), all of whom became worse while on Prozac. The behavioral abnormalities remained stable for weeks until the Prozac was reduced or stopped, and they were easily confused with the children's original emotional problems. Seven children on placebo developed no behavioral side effects.*

The Yale doctors did not present their findings at the FDA hearing.

Combined with Teicher's report on the disastrous Geller study, and with the growing anecdotal reports on Prozac abuse among young people, it becomes apparent that these drugs should not be given to children and youth. A drug's lack of proven efficacy in children, however, has never discouraged psychiatrists and pediatricians from liberally prescribing it. Neither has the inherent danger of exposing the growing brain to toxic substances. I was recently consulted in the case of a nine-year-old boy whose aggressivity markedly worsened on Prozac.

Gorman's Incidental Finding

As researchers combed the literature for evidence relevant to Prozac and behavioral abnormalities, others examined earlier studies in a new light.

In a 1987 Prozac study of panic disorder led by psychiatrist Jack Gorman from Columbia University, seven of sixteen patients dropped out due to "a cluster of symptoms characterized by increased agitation, restlessness, jitteriness, diarrhea, and insomnia." Two of these patients also developed depression and suicidal ideation on Pro-

---

*Despite the existence of data like this in the literature, psychiatrists make outlandish claims like the one captured in the headline, "Limited Data Suggest Fluoxetine Safe for Children," as reported in an article by Barbara Baker, 1993.

zac, one of them with no prior history of depression. The authors don't emphasize these threatening results.*

Muijen's Incidental Finding

In a 1988 study by M. Muijen from the Human Psychopharmacology Unit of the Medical College of St. Bartholomew's and the London Hospital, England, twelve of twenty-six Prozac patients dropped out because of side effects. Of these, two patients overdosed within two weeks of starting the study and had to be hospitalized due to "a deteriorating clinical state."†

Levine's Incidental Finding

In a 1987 Prozac trial for the treatment of obesity, Louise Levine from the Lilly Research Labs and her team noted that 7 percent of "non-depressed" patients developed depression during Prozac treatment. The information was elicited on "non-probing" inquiry and merely appears in a table.

The British Findings

The annual 1991 *British National Formulary*, a joint publication of the British Medical Association and the Royal Pharmaceutical Society of Great Britain, lists "suicidal ideation and violent behaviour" among the side effects of

---

*Remarkably, the Gorman study presented itself as confirming the usefulness of Prozac in panic disorder. But since it was not double-blind or placebo-controlled, it was worthless except for the frightening data on side effects.

†This study also found a statistically positive outcome for Prozac. This was accomplished by dropping the two suicide attempts from the study rather than including them as failures.

Prozac. One of the most prestigious journals in the world, Great Britain's *Lancet*, took a generally dim view of Prozac in an August 11, 1990, editorial.[70] Among the dangerous side effects of Prozac, *Lancet* included "the promotion of suicidal thoughts and behavior."

Evidence from a Medical Examiner's Office

In the March/April 1992 *Journal of Analytical Toxicology*, Robert O. Bost and Philip M. Kemp of the Southwestern Institute of Forensic Sciences reported on fifteen suicides in which Prozac or its metabolite was found in the body. The suicides, including ten by firearms, were evaluated by the medical examiner's office of Dallas County, Texas, over a nine-month period in 1990. In five cases there was data on the length of time Prozac was taken prior to the suicide: 5, 13, 16, and 35 days, and 3½ months. While there were also cases of suicide associated with other antidepressants, "the proportion taking fluoxetine and committing suicide is higher by an amount to be of concern to medical examiners and also to health care providers."

Bost and Kemp also report a new case of suicidal ideation in association with taking Prozac in a "weight-loss research program." They conclude, "All physicians who consider utilization of fluoxetine for their patients must be knowledgeable about this possible association and alerted to possible adverse effects in their patients."

A Unique Study of Patient Reports

In 1993, Seymour Fisher, Ph.D., Stephen Bryant, Pharm.D., and Thomas Kent, M.D., at the Department of Psychiatry at the University of Texas in Galveston published a study in the *Journal of Clinical Psychopharmacology* using patient reports of side effects made by a unique system. The outpatients phoned in adverse clinical events (ACEs) as soon as they happened, with special emphasis on new and unusual occurrences. The project compared Prozac with an older antidepressant, Desyrel (trazodone). The result indicated that Prozac causes "a higher incidence of various psychological/psychiatric ACEs including delusions and hallucinations, aggression, and suicidal ideation." The incidence rate for new suicidal ideation on the drug was a little less than one in one hundred patients (0.76 percent). Desyrel's rate was less than one-third that of Prozac's (0.25 percent). There were 2,487 patients in the Prozac group and they reported almost two-thirds of their side effects within the first two weeks of treatment.

What Does the Prozac Label Say About Drug-Induced Suicide and Violence?

Under "Precautions," the original Prozac label carried a general warning about the need to be aware of the danger of suicide before the antidepressant treatment has the time to take effect:

> *Suicide*—The possibility of a suicide attempt is inherent in depression and may persist until significant remission occurs. Close supervision of high-risk patients should accompany initial drug therapy. Prescriptions for Prozac should be written for the smallest quantity of capsules consistent with good patient management, in order to reduce the risk of overdose.

There is no hint in the "Precaution" that Prozac might cause or exacerbate suicidal tendencies. In a very misleading fashion, the statement directly suggests that treatment with Prozac can ultimately reduce the danger of suicide when there is no convincing evidence to support this hope.

Despite the flood of patient reports and independent

research studies linking Prozac to violence and suicide, Eli Lilly and the FDA have given only the most minimal recognition to the problem. In May 1990, "suicidal ideation" and "violent behaviors" became two of a dozen possible side effects added into a paragraph under "Postintroduction reports."* Any impact the paragraph might have is undermined by its introductory sentence describing the list of adverse reactions as based on "Voluntary reports of adverse events temporally associated with Prozac that have been received since market introduction and which may have no causal relationship with the drug . . ." Nothing further about suicide or violence has been added to the Prozac label since then.

AGITATION, STIMULATION, AND SUICIDE CAUSED BY PROZAC

In studies linking Prozac to violence against self and others, a number of clinical syndromes have been identified as causing the abnormal behavior or adding to the risk. We will now focus more closely on each of them.

As already illustrated in many cases and anecdotes throughout this book concerning both Prozac and the amphetamines, clinicians have noticed that agitation or anxiety can drive people to suicidal or violent actions.[71] At the FDA hearings, psychiatrist Jan Fawcett spoke on behalf of Eli Lilly, and reconfirmed the relationship.[72] He reviewed studies of suicide and concluded that anxiety, more than depression, predicts suicide within the year of its occurrence. In his own research, "[W]e found that anx-

---

*The adverse drug effects listed in the paragraph include cerebral vascular accident, confusion, dyskinesia, ecchymoses, gastrointestinal hemorrhage, hyperprolactinemia, pancreatitis, eosinophilic pneumonia, "suicidal ideation," thrombocytopenia, thrombocytopenic purpura, vaginal bleeding after drug withdrawal, and "violent behaviors."

iety, panic attacks, poor concentration, and insomnia formed a cluster which predicted suicide."[73]

These are precisely the stimulant adverse side effects most frequently produced by Prozac, pointing directly to how the drug increases the suicide risk in depressed patients by raising their level of anxiety or agitation. Fawcett did not make this point at the hearing, where it could have encouraged a label contrary to the aims of his sponsor, Eli Lilly. But Fawcett was well aware that Prozac agitation can precipitate suicide in depressed patients. He had already taken this position in the medical literature when discussing his research data on anxiety as a predictor of suicide. In a 1990 article, Fawcett wrote, "Suicide prevention is the first consideration in the treatment of major depression with anxiety." In the same paragraph, he recommended "aggressive treatment" with a sedative tranquilizer for patients with major depression if they "manifest risk factors for suicide, if the anxiety is severe or if the antidepressant selected causes jitteriness (fluoxetine). . . ."

Others have made the same recommendation: Prescribe additional sedatives to cut the risk of suicide and other adverse reactions to Prozac stimulation. The BGA, which plays a similar role in Germany to that of the FDA in the United States, required a Prozac label change in late 1989.* Under the category of "Risk Patients," the new label reads:

> Risk of Suicide: [Prozac] does not have a general sedative effect on the central nervous system. Therefore, for his/her own safety, the patient must be sufficiently observed, until the antidepressant effect of [Prozac] sets in. Taking an additional sedative may be necessary. This also applies in cases of extreme sleep disturbances or excitability.†

*In Germany, fluoxetine is called Fluctin. See Lily Deutschland Ltd., 1992.

†This is a certified translation by the Berlitz Translation Center of Woodland Hills, California.

The German label has another category of adverse reactions: "In addition, there are reports of the following health problems which occurred during treatment with [Prozac], although [Prozac] may not have been the cause." It lists "suicidal thoughts and aggressive behavior."

Without specifically mentioning the risk of suicide, the journal *Hospital Formulary* recognized that Prozac "causes significant agitation and restlessness in many patients that often require use of adjunctive sedating drugs."[74]

In reviewing the causes of drug-induced depression and suicide during the FDA hearings, Teicher observed that antidepressants as a class can precipitate episodes of mania or mania mixed with depression. Mixed mania and depression, he said, "carries a high risk for suicide. It is one of the most dangerous states a person can be in." Depressed patients who are lethargic and mentally sluggish, without being particularly suicidal, can be transformed by antidepressants into more high-energy suicide risks.[75]

By the time I began my training, psychiatrists were well aware that by "energizing" the still-depressed patient, antidepressants can facilitate suicide. Prozac, of course, is an especially energizing agent. Consultant Ida Hellander from the Public Citizen Research Group stressed at the FDA hearing that Prozac's side effects are "very different" from those of the tricyclics, and include "anxiety, insomnia, and agitation, and some restlessness." She pointed out that people driven by such painful emotions "can develop some desperate thoughts," including suicide. Another consultant, Regina Casper from the University of Chicago Department of Psychiatry, observed, "What we have heard this morning is that one of the side effects is the occurrence of agitation, of anxiety, of panic attacks, and of insomnia." Citing Fawcett's presentation on predictors of suicide, she expressed the need for further studies on the relationship between Prozac stimulation and suicide.

AKATHISIA, VIOLENCE, AND SUICIDE CAUSED BY PROZAC

We have seen that many cases of Prozac-induced violence and suicide involve agitation, anxiety, or panic. In many instances, the agitation probably stems from akathisia, a more specific drug-induced neurological reaction that can be difficult to distinguish from agitation. With agitation, anxiety, or panic, the psychological component dominates without an obvious physical manifestation in the form of hyperactivity. With akathisia, in addition to the inner tension or agitation, there is án accompanying compulsion to move the body, for example, by pacing, foot tapping, squirming about, or thrashing around in bed (see page 94).

Akathisia can drive people into actions destructive to themselves or others, including violence or suicide,[76] and even before the hearings, attention became focused on the fact that Prozac causes akathisia. Teicher and others at the FDA hearing did discuss akathisia as one of the possible causes of Prozac-induced violence and suicide; but Paul Leber, the FDA psychiatrist with the final say, stated that it did not matter if there were theoretical explanations of how Prozac might cause violence. Leber explained that the FDA was interested only in hard data proving that Prozac did in fact cause these behavioral aberrations.

In December 1991, with the FDA hearing two months past, Anthony Rothschild and Carol Locke, psychiatrists from McLean Hospital and Harvard Medical School, described three patients who made serious suicide attempts while suffering from Prozac-induced akathisia. In the first "rechallenge" study of Prozac's capacity to reproduce behavioral abnormalities a second time, the three patients were started once again on the drug under carefully monitored conditions. All three developed akathisia and again became suicidal. As one declared in retrospect, "I tried to kill myself because of these anxiety symptoms. It was not so much the depression."

Rothschild and Locke warned physicians to be alert to the fact that Prozac patients won't necessarily realize that their deterioration is drug induced. "Our patients had concluded their illness had taken such a dramatic turn for the worse that life was no longer worth living."[77]

In 1992 a Los Angeles psychiatric team led by William C. Wirshing described "five cases of what we think might be fluoxetine-induced akathisia accounting for suicidal ideation." The group included psychiatrist Theodore van Putten, one of the most thorough investigators of drug side effects in the world.

DEPRESSION AND APATHY CAUSED BY PROZAC

The concept that psychiatric medications can cause emotional disturbances, including depression and suicide, is not new or especially controversial within the profession. Clinical experience has repeatedly confirmed that many psychiatric drugs can cause depression. Reserpine, for example, is a potent neuroleptic drug, as well as an antihypertensive agent, whose use had to be curtailed because so many patients become depressed while taking it. The *Physicians' Desk Reference* carries warnings about the problem.

The Public Citizen Health Research Group in June 1990 discussed Prozac as a possible cause of depression and then listed fourteen other categories of drugs that can cause depression. A comprehensive list can be found in the notes section.[78]

Clinical Psychiatry News reporter Carl Sherman in 1994 interviewed experts and concluded, "The effects of drugs used to treat depression can mimic the symptoms the medications are intended to relieve." Sherman describes the views of well-known psychiatrist Donald F. Klein, director of research and therapeutics at the New York State Psychiatric Institute. Klein described the SSRIs as producing "lack of verve and spontaneity, passivity, apathy, and indifference."

Rudolf Hoehn-Saric and his colleagues from Johns Hopkins University Department of Psychiatry reported on six patients who developed apathy, indifference, and social withdrawal on Prozac and an as yet unapproved SSRI, fluvoxamine. One patient would complete tasks only if someone else structured them for her. She said, "This is what a frontal lobotomy must be like."

The symptoms of these patients *do* resemble those of people who have had a lobotomy. One patient lost her social judgment and wanted to serve cocktails in her bra "like Madonna" at a company party. Hoehn-Saric and his colleagues state that their patients displayed varying degrees of frontal-lobe dysfunction, including "apathy, flatness of affect [feeling] and lack of emotional concern, childishness and euphoria, socially inappropriate behavior, and difficulty foreseeing the outcome of an action." Typical of patients with frontal-lobe dysfunction, most did not appreciate their impairment.

I recently confirmed the same lobotomy-like effects in a woman in my practice who became increasingly apathetic, withdrawn, and depressed after several months on 100 mgs. per day of Zoloft. At first she rejected the idea that the drug was causing her deterioration, but she and her family recognized dramatic improvement within two or three days of stopping the medication.

The SSRI chemical-lobotomy syndrome is similar in appearance to the indifference produced by neuroleptics such as Haldol, Thorazine, Mellaril, and Prolixin. The neuroleptic or antipsychotic drugs are used primarily for the control of patients diagnosed as schizophrenic or acutely manic, and they produce an apathy or emotional flattening that makes these often-difficult patients more docile. The drugs produce this impact by directly interfering with dopamine, the major neurotransmitter from structures deeper in the brain to the frontal lobes.

Any gross interference with the frontal lobes "defuses" or deactivates patients, producing a robot-like state in which they are much less able to initiate activities. I have discussed this phenomenon in detail in several books and journal articles.[79]

The SSRIs also suppress dopamine neurotransmission to the frontal lobes, but they do so by a more indirect mechanism. When Prozac and other drugs stimulate the serotonergic system, dopamine tends to shut down as a compensatory reaction (see page 94). The effect is probably less complete and less consistent than that produced by the neuroleptics.

A SUMMARY OF HOW PROZAC CAN CAUSE VIOLENCE AND SUICIDE

Prozac can cause a range of psychological and neurological disorders that can lead to destructive actions.

First, Prozac frequently causes *agitation, panic, or anxiety*. These emotional responses can make a person desperate enough to commit suicide or to perpetrate violence.

Second, Prozac causes *mania* in a significant percentage of patients, and mania can lead to suicide and violence. *Euphoria*, which is common on Prozac, can be viewed as mild or incipient mania.

Third, Prozac very commonly causes the neurological disorder *akathisia*, which can drive people into violence toward themselves or others.

These first three drug-induced disorders—agitation, mania, and akathisia—can be difficult to distinguish from each other. Together, they are the most commonly associated syndromes with Prozac-induced violence and suicide, as well as other bizarre and destructive actions. This is consistent with the known effects of amphetamines, which produce similar stimulant syndromes and behavioral abnormalities. As Teicher and others described at the FDA hearing, drug-induced stimulation can also increase the person's energy level and hence his or her capacity to carry out actions. The still-depressed person is thus enabled to act on destructive impulses.

Fourth, Prozac can cause *depression* or symptoms that mimic depression—including fatigue, agitation, social withdrawal, emotional flatness or apathy, loss of appetite, loss of sexual desire or capacity, and loss of loving connection to other people. Prozac users may actually become depressed or may simply think they are more depressed, which often adds up to the same thing. Either state can lead to suicidal ruminations and actions. Withdrawal from Prozac can also produce depression or related symptoms, including most of the responses categorized under major depression, such as suicidal tendencies.

Fifth, Prozac can cause *paranoia*—an irrational fear and blaming of others—than can lead to violence against others, and, less commonly, against oneself.

Sixth, Prozac can increase *obsessive-compulsive* thoughts and behavior, including preoccupations with death, murder, and suicide.

Seventh, Prozac frequently causes *insomnia*, and sleeplessness can drive people to despair and sometimes to suicide.[80]

There is another tragic way in which Prozac can lead to despair and suicide. When patients are told that they are being given the benefit of the latest miracle cure, it can set them up for a potentially fatal emotional letdown. As many such victims have told me, "When even the drugs didn't work on me, I figured I was a lost cause." People who have lost their "last hope" are especially prone to suicide.

BIOCHEMICAL CAUSES OF SSRI-INDUCED VIOLENCE AND SUICIDE

Given all the evidence that Prozac does cause violence against self and others, is there a known pharmacological mechanism to account for it?

The most widely accepted of all theories in biological psychiatry is the sluggish serotonin theory of impulsivity. There are hundreds of research papers and reviews that claim to substantiate it.[81] Briefly, the theory says that reduced serotonergic neurotransmission causes "loss of impulse control," leading to murder, suicide, and other out-of-control behaviors, such as hyperactivity in children and delinquency in teenagers. Remarkably, depression is also attributed to the same sluggish serotonin, although its inclusion within the concept of impulsivity requires a stretch of the imagination.

The sluggish serotonin theory has gained so much support that government scientists have become increasingly vocal in using it to explain vast social problems, such as violence in America,[82] and some of the media, eager for biological explanations of violence, have embraced these claims.[83]

From early on, researchers at Eli Lilly used the sluggish serotonin theory to justify the development and marketing of Prozac and other SSRIs. In theory, the SSRIs are supposed to fire up (just as someone might stoke a fading fire) serotonergic neurotransmission, overcoming any inherent sluggishness in the system.

But to the extent that the sluggish serotonin theory is true, then Prozac is a menace. While Prozac is trying to stimulate or energize serotonin activity by blocking the removal of the neurotransmitter from its synapse, the brain is trying to compensate by shutting down the nerves that produce the serotonin. When Prozac blocks the removal of serotonin from the synapse, causing an excess

amount of it to remain there, the brain cell reacts by re-
fusing to release any additional serotonin into the synapse.[84] These compensatory mechanisms are especially
active in the first two weeks of drug treatment and the-
oretically could cause a net decrease in serotonergic activity at that time.

The initial compensatory shutdown mechanism is not
the only way the brain tries to overcome the Prozac-
induced glut of serotonin in the synapses. The brain develops another more ominous reaction that continues to
increase over time. The second mechanism—called down-
regulation—causes receptors for serotonin literally to disappear from the brain. As discussed in chapter 4, in many
areas in the brains of experimental animals, the receptors
drastically diminish in number, sometimes with losses as
high as 40 percent and 60 percent in regions of the brain
involved in mental functioning.[85] The changes are persistent during exposure to the drug. Since no trace of the
receptors can be found, the most likely assumption is that
they have died off.*

Are these serotonin receptor losses permanent? Are
patients taking Prozac at risk of losing large percentages
of their brain receptors? The straightforward studies required to determine the permanency of receptor losses
are not being carried out. I've seen no indication that Lilly
has made any attempt to see if the receptor losses are
permanent. Although they would be extremely easy and
inexpensive to do in the early stages of animal testing, the
FDA has not asked the drug companies to carry them out
as a prerequisite for the approval of psychiatric drugs. In

---

*Diagram A on page 21 shows the serotonin synapse and mechanism
whereby Prozac blocks the removal of serotonin from its synapse. As
a glut of serotonin develops, receptors on the presynaptic nerve cause
it to shut down or put out smaller amounts of serotonin. These receptors are not depicted. Notice the many serotonin receptors on the postsynaptic nerve waiting for serotonin to connect with them to fire the
nerve. When there's a glut of serotonin in the synapse, these begin to
disappear.

recent interviews with neuroscientists around the country, I have found no inclination on the part of any of them to investigate whether or not these changes in the brain can become permanent.

One highly respected psychiatrist and laboratory researcher who is a university professor recently told me that a finding of irreversible receptor loss could be used against Eli Lilly in lawsuits. If there is a permanent reduction in the numbers of serotonin receptors, then permanent serotonergic sluggishness could set in, with the predicted result of increased impulsive behavior.* Nonetheless, the researcher went on to say that he thought such studies were not worth doing. When specifically asked, he confirmed that he, like many others in the field, receives funding from Eli Lilly for his own receptor studies.

Work with much less complex receptors and synapses in rat muscle confirms our apprehension about the ultimate fate of disappearing receptors. Research reported at the 1994 meetings of the American Association for the Advancement of Science (AAAS) by physician-researcher Jeff Lichtman of Washington University has demonstrated that large-scale receptor losses can become permanent with the eventual loss of the synapses themselves.[86]

It seems possible that patients taking antidepressant drugs, perhaps for only weeks or months, are suffering widespread permanent losses of brain receptors and synapses. The tendency of the drug effect to wear off for some patients—the development of so-called immunity—

---

*The serotonin system requires not only a nerve to produce and release the neurotransmitter, but also a second (postsynaptic) nerve to receive it (see diagram on page 25). With a permanent decline in the number of receptors, the second nerve would be less able to receive stimulation. This sluggishness would become especially apparent over time or once the Prozac had been stopped, leaving the brain with no serotonergic drug stimulation and fewer receptors to receive whatever serotonin was being naturally released.

may reflect receptor loss. The development of depression or impulsive behavior may be another result.

Since most antidepressants block the reuptake of neurotransmitters, with the subsequent disappearance of many receptors,[87] permanent receptor loss may occur with most of these drugs. It could be worse with SSRIs because of the intensity with which they overstimulate serotonergic nerves.

Because the receptor losses occur in areas that regulate intellectual and emotional life, there is literally no telling what the permanent impact on each person's mind will be. It is reprehensible that Eli Lilly and other drug companies have not studied this danger on their own. It is disgraceful that the FDA and the medical profession have not required these studies prior to drug approval or at any time thereafter.

LILLY RESEARCHERS DEFEND PROZAC

Although Lilly researchers seemingly have never raised the problem of Prozac-induced sluggish serotonin,[88] I am not alone in suggesting that it might cause murderous or suicidal compulsions. Several researchers, including North Carolina psychiatrist C. Thomas Gualtieri, have mentioned the possible connection between Prozac-induced reductions in serotonergic activity and suicidal or violent behavior.[89] In defending against the accusation, Lilly investigators Ray Fuller and Charles Beasley claim that the overall effect of Prozac is to put the brain into a *better* balance and that no parts of the brain suffer from sluggish serotonin during the process of compensatory shutdown and down-regulation with the loss of receptors.[90] Yet some research does indicate that the system can at times become sluggish as a result of Prozac.[91]

Remember that Prozac was rationalized as a treatment on the grounds that overly impulsive people have sluggish serotonin as demonstrated by the relatively low amounts of 5-HIAA, the serotonin breakdown product, in their brain and spinal fluid. But Prozac does not raise 5-HIAA; it reduces it.[92] The Lilly researchers try to show that, despite this, the serotonergic nerves are firing more strongly than ever, but this is conjectural. There's no way to measure the levels of serotonin nerve activity throughout the brain at all times, and all the relevant research is conducted using animals who have far less complex brains than humans.

In the midst of denying that Prozac can cause serotonergic sluggishness, the Lilly researchers, Fuller and Beasley, do admit that if Prozac did sometimes produce sluggishness, "it might explain the behavior observed by these authors," that is, compulsive suicidality.

THE FINAL FDA COMMITTEE VOTE

Despite their biases and conflicts of interest, several committee members and consultants favored adding a warning to Prozac's label that would alert physicians to the *possibility* that Prozac and other antidepressants might precipitate suicide. But the chairman of the committee, Casey, as well as Leber from the FDA, were against it.

Committee member James Claghorn, medical director of Clinical Research Associates in Houston, Texas, specifically suggested the following addition to the label: "In a small number of patients, depressive symptoms have worsened during therapy, including the emergence of suicidal thoughts and attempts. Surveillance throughout treatment is recommended." Despite pressure from Casey and Leber, three of the nine members voted for a modification. That one-third of the committee would take such a position is, in our opinion, an indicator of the strength of the evidence.

WHAT'S GOING ON HERE?

So, why hasn't Eli Lilly faced the dangers of Prozac? How could the FDA—and a majority of its psychopharmacology committee—exonerate the drug in regard to suicide and violence? How and why do organized psychiatry, Eli Lilly, and the FDA turn a blind eye to warnings raised in 1991 in my own book, *Toxic Psychiatry*, as well as in the publications of the teams led by Martin Teicher at Harvard, by Robert King at Yale, and by W. Creaney from North Wales? How can they ignore the warnings voiced by Anthony Rothschild and Carol Locke at Harvard and by C. Thomas Gualtieri at Chapel Hill, North Carolina, as well as other clinicians and researchers? How do they dismiss concerns raised by sources as divergent as the *Lancet* of Great Britain and Nader's Public Citizen Health Research Group? How do they ignore the existence of the national Prozac Survivors Support Group with its hundreds of members, as well as the poignant presentations at the FDA hearings by individual citizens and their families, and the record-breaking numbers of adverse reaction reports received by the agency regarding Prozac? How do they rationalize away the growing number of reports in the literature, the unprecedented number of anecdotal stories in the media, and the tidal wave of lawsuits generated by injured Prozac survivors and their families?

The answer to these questions lies in the intricate web of connections among the FDA, the drug companies, and the psychiatric community. This psycho-pharmaceutical complex is the subject of the following chapter.

EIGHT

Pushing Drugs in America

The Long Financial Tentacles of Eli Lilly

When the cigarette company Philip Morris Inc. was recently accused of stifling a study that showed nicotine to be addictive, few people were disillusioned or even surprised. The American Tobacco Institute, funded by the cigarette companies, has become a symbol of self-interested scientific analysis as it has tried to deny the association between smoking and cancer. The FDA is currently taking the position that nicotine is so addictive that it should be regulated by the agency, and of course everyone knows that the cigarette industry will resist this conclusion.

Despite the public and the media's relative sophistication about cigarette company claims for scientific objectivity about its nonprescription drug nicotine, they often assume that the manufacturers of prescription drugs will conduct themselves by higher ethical and scientific standards. But do they?

HOW ADVERSE DRUG REACTIONS ARE REPORTED TO AND EVALUATED BY THE FDA

It is generally agreed that the premarketing studies done by drug companies for the FDA cannot adequately detect many serious adverse reactions and that a very substantial number of potentially dangerous drugs continue to slip through the approval process.[1]

The scientifically controlled premarketing studies, averaging four to six weeks in length, are much too short to pick up most risks. The individual studies at specific sites typically involve fewer than one hundred patients, so that even serious effects that occur at a rate of one in one hundred are likely to be missed. Yet once the drug is marketed to the public, a rate of one in one hundred adverse reactions adds up to ten thousand victims among the first one million patients.

In discussing adverse drug reactions in chapter 4, we looked at the limitations inherent in the premarketing studies, including the small size of the sample and the relatively brief duration of the controlled studies. We also pointed out that many serious side effects are not discovered until after the marketing of a drug has begun.

To detect postmarketing risks, the FDA relies upon a spontaneous report system based on voluntary reports from physicians who take the time to send a report to the drug company or the FDA. This process is informal and voluntary. Up to 40 percent of physicians do not even realize that the FDA reporting system exists.[2] You may have to tell your own doctor how to send in an adverse drug reaction report (see Appendix for materials).

Critics of the FDA,[3] as well as FDA officials I have interviewed, agree that the postmarketing surveillance for adverse drug effects is very inadequate.* Congress and the public, FDA officials explained to me, have wanted the FDA to emphasize the initial approval process with resultant neglect of more long-term monitoring of adverse drug reactions.

Eli Lilly, like all drug companies, is required within fifteen days to report to the FDA any information it receives about serious adverse reactions not already

---

*In chapter 4, some aspects of postmarketing surveillance are discussed.

sufficiently described in its official label.* Only a small fraction of serious drug side effects ever get reported to the manufacturer or the FDA, yet in the case of Prozac, the FDA has now received more than 28,000 adverse reaction reports of all kinds since the drug became available in January 1988. This is far more than for any other drug in FDA history.[4] During the late 1980s and early 1990s, the vast majority of these reports came through the drug companies before being sent to the FDA. Therefore, Lilly's method of handling the reports is critical.

During the 1991 FDA Prozac hearing, Bruce Stadel from the FDA's Division of Epidemiology and Surveillance made a presentation on behalf of the agency. Stadel has both medical and public health degrees, and he was clearly not satisfied with the way the FDA collected its data on adverse drug reactions.

Stadel summarized data showing that the FDA had received 880 spontaneous reports of adverse reactions to Prozac in the combined categories of suicide *attempt* (not suicidal thoughts), overdose, and psychotic depression.[5] There were no duplications in this final tally.

Because of the reports by Teicher, King, and others (see chapter 7), the public and the FDA were especially concerned about drug-induced compulsive or violent suicidal *ideation*—thoughts or feelings that were not carried into action. Suicidal actions are too infrequent for accurate estimates of their rates in relatively small populations, but suicidal ideations are much more common, and were reported in several Prozac studies. Why did the

---

*By law, all drug companies are required to notify the FDA within fifteen days of any serious, new adverse drug reactions, or of a marked increase in the reported rate of recognized serious side effects. More routine reports of side effects must also be sent to the FDA but they are sent in periodically as a group. While the label for Prozac acknowledges the existence of reports of suicidality in association with the drug, it specifically states that no causality has been proven. Therefore, reports of drug-related suicidality or suicide must be reported within fifteen days to the FDA.

FDA have no data on this all-important phenomena from its spontaneous reporting system?

LILLY HIDES PROZAC-INDUCED SUICIDAL IDEATION

Most adverse drug reaction reports are received by the FDA on special forms submitted by the drug companies and then entered into the agency's computerized system. Items can be logged in the FDA computer only according to a fixed list of terms. After 1989, drug-induced suicidal *acts* were included in the FDA's system of codification; but to this day, the FDA does not have a specific category for drug-induced suicidal *ideation*.

Stadel admitted that the FDA's system placed limitations on the usefulness of its data in evaluating Prozac's potential to cause suicidal ideation and acts. He also knew, but did not mention, that Eli Lilly's system also lacks a category for suicidal ideation.* When a doctor sends in an adverse drug reaction report to Lilly that includes suicide ideation, Lilly lists it under something else.

I had my own dismaying encounter with Lilly's system of codifying adverse drug reactions. On February 24, 1993, I sent the drug company a copy of my published medical report on Catherine, a young woman hospitalized for suicidal feelings brought about by taking Prozac.[6] The title of the article was "A Case of Fluoxetine-Induced Stimulant Side Effects with Suicidal Ideation Associated with a Possible Withdrawal Reaction ('Crashing')." The title made clear that drug-induced *suicidal ideation* was central to the report, and I drew attention to it in the cover letter as well.

Lilly sent me back a copy of their filing of my report with the FDA, containing a list of terms that were sup-

---

*Our information on Lilly's coding system is current as of early 1993. We do not know if changes have been made since that time.

posed to describe Catherine's adverse reaction to Prozac; but the list did not include anything about suicidal thoughts or feelings. It did indicate "depression" as one of the drug side effects, along with more than a dozen others, including tremor, insomnia, abnormal vision, paranoid reaction, and addiction. Suicidal ideation was mentioned in the "free text"—a written paragraph that accompanies the list of terms—but nothing in that text gets listed in the FDA's computer.

In a telephone interview with me on March 16, 1994, the FDA's Bruce Stadel confirmed that FDA computers cannot pull up the text that comes along with drug company's reports. In evaluating Eli Lilly's adverse reaction reports for his presentation at the hearing, for example, Stadel relied solely on the computer printout. Since neither the FDA nor Eli Lilly has any category for suicidal ideation, there was no direct evidence bearing upon one of the key issues at the hearing.

After I received a copy of Lilly's report to the FDA, I wrote back to the drug company and requested that they list suicidal ideation as an adverse event from my case. Lilly never responded. My reporting to Lilly on Prozac-induced suicidal ideation was futile.

By not recognizing suicidal ideation as a category in its list of possible Prozac-induced adverse effects, Lilly has protected itself from producing any data that could incriminate the drug. Lilly continued with this practice despite the professional and public demand for specific data on Prozac-induced suicidal ideation during the controversy that led up to the 1991 FDA hearings and thereafter.

I sent a copy of my Prozac case to the FDA as well as to Eli Lilly. The FDA's handling of the two reports—one from me and one from the drug company—itself raises questions. The FDA computerized system lists only four adverse drug reactions from my report: depression, insomnia, no drug effect, and personality disorder. Not only is suicidal ideation left out, but so also are three key elements that suggest Prozac is a potential drug of abuse. Mentioned by Lilly, but not by the FDA, are withdrawal syndrome, tolerance increase, and addiction. If a question is raised about Prozac's potential for abuse, the FDA has ruled out access to all the information on the subject that I submitted to them directly as well as through Eli Lilly.

THE RATE OF PROZAC-RELATED VIOLENCE WAS HIGHER, BUT NEVER MIND

In reviewing the FDA's data during the 1991 hearing, Stadel did find a disproportionately high number of spontaneous reports of Prozac-induced "hostility and intentional injury" during the first year of the drug's marketing, followed by a "major take-off" in reported incidents after the publicity surrounding Teicher's report from Harvard and the Wesbecker multiple-murder case (p. 148). This was a critical finding—an unexpectedly large number of reports of violence. Stadel mentioned this all-important fact in passing and then immediately stopped his slide presentation and went on to a more general discussion.[7]

Remarkably, no FDA committee members or consultants asked Stadel for more specific information or challenged him about glossing over one of the major issues of the hearing—increased reported rates of violence due to Prozac. Stadel himself told me in the telephone interview that he could not recall the data and had left it behind in his transfer to another division at the FDA.

The FDA spontaneous reporting system has limited utility. It can best be used as a signal that an adverse reaction exists rather than as a measure of its actual frequency. Corroborating evidence is usually required to prove a causal connection between the drug and the reported adverse reaction. Nonetheless, the spontaneous reporting system can provide such a powerful signal. These signals have resulted on many occasions in the FDA requiring a label change or even the withdrawal of a drug from the market. It's a shame that Eli Lilly and the FDA have crippled the system in regard to its capacity to detect one of the most important adverse reactions of all—suicidal ideation.

THE MEDICAL-INDUSTRIAL COMPLEX

Why doesn't the FDA, the medical profession, or someone in the health field make a big fuss about these and other obviously negligent acts and attitudes within the drug industry?

The "Medical-Industrial Complex"[8] has once again come under criticism in the debate over health care, but the nation has little idea how much raw power is exerted by these interests throughout American society. In *Toxic Psychiatry* I drew attention to one particular segment, the psycho-pharmaceutical complex. It includes private pharmaceutical companies, government agencies such as the FDA and NIH, professional organizations such as the American Psychiatric Association, psychiatric departments in hospitals and medical schools, insurance companies, and even private philanthropic organizations such as the National Association for Mental Health and the MacArthur Foundation. Recently, so-called parent groups like NAMI (National Alliance for the Mentally Ill) and CH.A.D.D. (Children with Attention-Deficit Disorders) have become politically involved.[9] They lobby side by side with organized psychiatry to push biological theories and drugs for the control of their children.

Sometimes there are flashes of competition among various interests in the psycho-pharmaceutical complex—for example, insurance companies sometimes try to cut the costs of psychiatric treatment and the FDA sometimes exerts itself against industry on behalf of consumer safety. But by and large, their major efforts go toward supporting the biological model of human suffering and the dispensing of pills as a solution.

The members of the psycho-pharmaceutical complex tend to enjoy one seamless cooperative enterprise, fueled by billions of dollars from the drug companies, as well as funds from government agencies and private sources. This was amply demonstrated at the 1991 FDA hearings where the majority of committee members and official consultants enjoyed ties to the drug companies.

Whose Side Is the FDA On?

While many Americans, including physicians, believe that the FDA takes tough stands toward the pharmaceutical industry, this has never been so. As medical writer Morton Mintz documented thirty years ago in *The Therapeutic Nightmare*, from the beginning the FDA has more often failed than succeeded in its mission.* To this day, the FDA continues to draw criticism from Congress and elsewhere for everything from taking bribes and courting the favor of drug companies to withholding lifesaving drugs from the public.[10]

The continuing problem is described in a recent story in the *AARP Bulletin* that begins, "Stepped-up industry pressure and election-year politics are driving the Food and Drug Administration (FDA) to back away rapidly from some consumer protection policies it favored as recently as last fall, consumer advocates charge."[11] In yet another recent criticism of the FDA from the House Government Operations Committee, Representative Donald M. Payne (D-NJ) declared, "Patients trust the FDA to protect them, but under the deregulation fever of the last 12 years, that has not always happened."[12]

*For example, Mintz describes the thalidomide disaster in the early 1960s in which a sleeping pill given to pregnant women caused hundreds of deformed babies in Europe and a lesser number in America. Both industry and the FDA resisted efforts to alert the American public and the medical profession to the danger, even after it became apparent in Europe.

Recent scandals over the minor tranquilizer Halcion have further exposed the FDA's lax and supportive attitude toward the pharmaceutical industry. Banned in England because, among other things, it can produce paranoia and violence, Halcion remains approved in the United States.[13] As I have documented in detail, the maker of Halcion, Upjohn, is one of the most generous drug companies when it comes to making huge donations to organized psychiatry in the United States.[14] In the middle of the flap over Halcion, I disclosed that Upjohn had given the American Psychiatric Association $1.5 million in cash to use as it pleased.[15] In response to my criticism, both the American Psychiatric Association and Upjohn wrote letters praising their mutual "partnership."[16]

The problem, from the beginning, has been simple enough. The bureaucratic regulators end up feeling much more cozy with the regulated than with the consumer. On one side of the equation, the regulators are being courted, educated, lobbied, politically threatened, cajoled, and flattered by big industry, their full-time lobbyists, their paid scientists, and their financially beholden representatives in Congress and the government. Even outright bribery can take place.[17] On the other side of the equation, there's the consumer, inadequately funded, poorly organized, incompletely informed, ill-represented, and often working on a part-time volunteer basis. It's not much of a contest when it comes to influencing the regulators.

Enormous amounts of money are required to process a drug through the FDA and the potential profits are astronomical. One former FDA official told me that the cost of the approval process can run into the "hundreds of millions" for one drug. He estimated that Lilly spent $80 million getting Prozac through the FDA. With such a huge investment at stake, and with the prospect of billions in profits, enormous pressure can be brought upon the FDA to find a way to approve a drug.

A Window into Leber's Attitudes

In our excursion into the FDA Prozac hearing, we found that the "watchdog" agency seemed more intent on watching over the interests of drug companies than those of the consumer. After the tragic stories were presented, and before the committee heard any scientific evidence, the FDA's Paul Leber declared there was insufficient evidence for the claim that Prozac could cause destructive behavior. The committee chair, psychiatrist Daniel Casey, announced his own similar position. Those opinions would have seemed compelling to many committee members. Casey was the committee chair, and Leber is director of the Division of Neuropharmacological Drug Products and the man responsible for appointing them.

We get a window into Leber's philosophy from his handling of tardive dyskinesia, the permanent neurological disorder produced by neuroleptic drugs such as Thorazine, Mellaril, Navane, Prolixin, and Haldol, and the worst drug-induced disaster in the history of medicine (see my book *Toxic Psychiatry* for details). On January 31, 1985, Leber convened the 27th meeting of the Pharmacological Drugs Advisory Committee to obtain advisory committee approval for a label change—a uniform warning for tardive dyskinesia to be required of all the companies manufacturing or distributing neuroleptic drugs. By then, the neuroleptics had been in use for more than three decades.

As we noted in chapter 4, tardive dyskinesia occurs at the astronomical rate of approximately 5 percent per year in neuroleptic-treated patients. Among older individuals, including hundreds of thousands of elderly residents of nursing homes, 20 percent will develop tardive dyskinesia during each year of exposure. Tardive dyskinesia is a medically caused catastrophe that has victimized tens of millions of people in the past four decades.

Why, after thirty years, did Leber's division of the FDA finally at last insist upon a uniform *warning* in every manufacturer's label? Was it an increased ethical, medical, or scientific awareness?

It snowed on that day in January 1985 in Rockville, Maryland,* and because of the bad weather, a quorum could not be achieved. So the meeting became a less formal "workshop" in which Leber seemed to speak with unusual freedom about his division's relationship with the drug companies.

Leber explained that he himself initially resisted the idea of a uniform warning on tardive dyskinesia because he thought the existing labels were adequate. Thus, he explained, he was "somewhat surprised, in the fall of 1983, that we heard a clamor from the press, from the public media, that the products marketed as neuroleptics, largely antipsychotics, were not adequately labeled. . . ."† The publicity led the FDA to decide "to err on the side of giving overt statements of warning rather than assuming what seemed very clear." In other words, against his own judgment, Leber gave in to public pressure.

At the January 31, 1985, meeting of the Psychopharmacologic Drugs Advisory Committee, Leber further elaborated on how his division of the FDA had been working closely with industry for one and one-half years to develop new tardive dyskinesia guidelines "that would be fair and that would be acceptable to everyone." The proposed label had been sent back and forth between Leber and the corporations, with Leber modifying it to their

---

*The headquarters of the FDA, in the suburbs outside Washington, D.C.
†That "clamor" in the fall of 1983 was caused by the publication of my medical book, *Psychiatric Drugs: Hazards to the Brain*, and related reform efforts by our Center for the Study of Psychiatry Network. Prepublication, I shared the manuscript with a network TV producer and it resulted on November 28 to 30, 1983, in a three-part series by Dan Rather, "Prescription for Despair," on the CBS Evening News, as well as other media. The problem of tardive dyskinesia grows, but with relatively little recent media interest.

desires, until they agreed with the final result. That final result, needless to say, was even weaker than the one originally proposed by his division.

Leber called this "due process." But it was a process that lacked the participation of consumer- or patient-oriented groups, or any other watchdog groups. No one devoted to patient or consumer advocacy and no one critical of industry was involved. Leber's due process involved writing a warning that was "acceptable" to industry.

Leber put it this way: "We needed equitable labeling that did not cause injury to industry, as much as it should not cause injury to patients or physicians who have to use neuroleptics under trying circumstances." But there is no mandate from Congress requiring the FDA to "not cause injury to industry" or to protect industry "as much as" patients or physicians. There's no Congressional mandate to protect physicians, either. The FDA's mandate is to protect patients and consumers.

If the FDA carried out its mandate to protect consumers, then some corporations and some physicians would inevitably at times feel injured, especially in their pocketbooks. That's the whole point of the FDA function: To force industry to meet standards with which industry and the medical profession, left to their own interests, would not comply.

Leber's commitment not to hurt industry added up to accommodating industry. The uniform label for tardive dyskinesia, created by agreement between the FDA and industry, remains woefully inadequate. For example, it gives no hint of the incredibly high incidence of the disorder or the huge numbers of people afflicted by it. It does not mention that many TD patients develop mental disabilities, including dementia.

Leber's selection of Daniel Casey to be chairman of the Psychopharmacological Drugs Committee during the period covering the 1991 Prozac hearing indicates his continued tendency to favor industry. Casey was also present at the FDA's 1985 tardive dyskinesia workshop. In the incestuous world of drug experts, Casey was at that time acting as a paid consultant to McNeil, the manufacturer of Haldol, a neuroleptic with some of the most extreme neurological side effects. Over the years, Casey has taken controversial stances on TD that have helped to protect doctors and drug companies from criticism and from lawsuits.*

Conflict of Interest on the FDA Advisory Committee

The FDA has 41 advisory committees that have no inherent power, but whose nonbinding recommendations lend credibility to the FDA decision-making process. The members of the psychopharmacological review committee are appointed from outside the agency for fixed three-year terms.

The FDA review committee system has recently come under criticism because many of its advisors, who are supposed to have expertise in specific areas, often have ties to industry and a vested professional interest in the very treatments they are evaluating.[18] This turned out to be true about the advisory committee, as well as the consultants, at the 1991 FDA Prozac hearing.

In addition to chairman Daniel Casey, the FDA's psychopharmacology committee and its consultants consisted of fifteen members, nearly all of them psychiatrists. As psychiatrists, they were wholly committed to maintaining the good name of their profession and its treatments.

*In a tardive dyskinesia malpractice suit in Alaska (Novelli, 1991), I was a medical expert for the plaintiff (a tardive dyskinesia patient) and Casey was a medical expert for the defendant (a state hospital and its doctors). Casey testified that giving the offending neuroleptic drug to the patient, who already had tardive dyskinesia, did not make her disorder worse or reduce the eventual likelihood of remission. I testified that continuing to give her the drug caused a permanent worsening in her condition. The jury found for the patient and awarded her damages.

They would be very reluctant to reach conclusions that might lead to public condemnation and massive lawsuits against the profession and its benefactor drug companies.

There were no unequivocal consumer advocates* in the process and, in fact, the FDA relates almost entirely to drug companies and organized psychiatry, to the exclusion of the consumers it is mandated to serve.

Most shocking, many members of this group of FDA-chosen advisors had so many financial ties to drug companies that the FDA felt compelled to address the problem. The FDA's official "Conflict of Interest Statement" at the 1991 Prozac hearing declared that the meeting would entail "no specific issues dealing with a specific product or sponsor drug company." Since no particular drug or company would be the focus of the meeting—but rather the general question of antidepressants, violence, and suicide—the agency wouldn't disqualify anyone. This was a simple ruse to avoid having to disqualify anyone with connections to the companies that make SSRIs, especially Eli Lilly. Except for Lilly, whose drug Prozac held the center of attention throughout the day, every other company invited by the FDA to make a presentation in fact declined to show up.

The FDA ended up giving *five of nine committee members* "waivers" to participate.†[19] As one example, FDA

---

*Physician Ida Hellander was present as a consultant from the Public Citizen Health Research Group, a Nader-related organization headed by Sidney Wolfe, M.D. While on occasion critical of the overuse of drugs, Wolfe is basically an advocate for them. Wolfe does not work with reform organizations representing consumers such as the National Association of Psychiatric Survivors or the Prozac Survivors Support Group (see Appendix). He collaborates closely with E. Fuller Torrey, one of the most radically biological and prodrug psychiatrists in the country.

†Receiving waivers were committee members James Claghorn, M.D.; David Dunner, M.D.; Jeffrey Lieberman, M.D.; Robert Hamer, M.D.; Lin Keh-Ming, M.D.; and consultant Michael Stanley, Ph.D. For the list and brief explanations, see Food and Drug Administration, September 20, 1991B.

committee member James L. Claghorn, M.D., is Medical Director of Clinical Research Associates of Houston, Texas, a firm that is conducting research on the SSRI Paxil (paroxetine) for SmithKline Beecham. Claghorn himself is principle investigator on a grant from Sandoz, the manufacturer of the tricyclic antidepressant Pamelor (nortriptyline). Not disclosed in the waiver signed by Claghorn and the FDA, Claghorn was a clinical investigator for Lilly in one of the Prozac trials.

As another example, disclosed in a September 13, 1991, FDA memorandum, committee member Jeffrey Lieberman, M.D., Director of Research at Hillside Hospital in Glen Oaks, New York, and a professor at the Albert Einstein College of Medicine in New York, was a principle investigator for several grants from Sandoz, and gave paid lectures sponsored by the company.

Michael E. Stanley, Ph.D., professor of clinical psychopharmacology at Columbia's College of Physicians and Surgeons, was a consultant to the FDA at the hearings. Stanley's potential conflicts of interest are described in a September 17, 1991, FDA memorandum. His duties at Columbia involved him in many drug company research projects, including two grants from Pfizer for testing the SSRI Zoloft (sertraline). But most remarkable is Stanley's personal financial relationship with Eli Lilly. At the time of the FDA hearing, Stanley was being paid $26,250 by Eli Lilly to write a paper on the very subject of the hearing—"examining the possible relationship between suicidal behavior, treatment with antidepressants, and serotonergic systems." Lilly would not pay so much money without anticipating a favorable result.

Paul Leber and the FDA knowingly hired Stanley as a virtual double agent, working for both the FDA and Lilly at the same time on the same controversial issue. The FDA's use of him as a consultant at the Prozac hearing indicates a callous disregard for the very concept of conflict of interest.

Perhaps an even more disturbing conflict of interest involved committee member David Dunner, a psychiatrist from the University of Washington Medical Center in Seattle.[20] Dunner is actively involved in obtaining grants for the university and in administering them as the chief investigator, although he himself is paid by salary from the university. In addition to $500,000 worth of drug company grants that he supervises at his university, there was, at the time of the FDA hearing, $200,000 in grants "pending" from Eli Lilly, including one for an antidepressant study.

The September 16, 1991, FDA summary of Dunner's financial relationships states that he "anticipates doing occasional lecturing" for about ten drug companies. In reality, he had already done at least several dozen paid lectures for Eli Lilly alone. Although we don't have specific information on how much he was paid for these drug company–sponsored presentations, the "honoraria" usually run at least $1,000 apiece, plus lavish expenses.

The FDA description of Dunner's activities did not mention that he had been a principal investigator in one of the studies, Protocol 27, used by Lilly to gain FDA approval of Prozac (see chapter 3).

A year before the hearing, Dunner had given a presentation at a workshop for doctors on depression sponsored by Eli Lilly. A report on his presentation in *Psychiatric Times* describes Dunner as citing Teicher's study on intense and violent suicidal thoughts in response to Prozac.[21] The report, summarizing Dunner's remarks, states, "While there is no evidence from controlled studies to support these findings, close clinical monitoring is advisable."

It would have been helpful if Dunner had taken that position at the FDA hearings. (If the FDA had required a statement about the need for "close clinical monitoring" concerning Prozac-induced suicide, it could have saved many lives.) But the hearing record shows that Dunner made no such comments. He left early, leaving behind a proxy to vote negatively on the question of whether or not there is any "credible evidence" to conclude that antidepressants can cause or intensify suicidal thoughts.

It is difficult to decide what is more reprehensible—FDA consultants and voting committee members so beholden to drug companies that they could not possibly make an objective evaluation or laboratory researchers so dependent upon the same drug companies that they cannot carry out objective research. What is clear is the iron grip that the drug companies hold on every aspect of the mental health profession, from the labs to the clinical offices, and beyond to the FDA itself.

Although the FDA has been generous in allowing experts with drug industry ties and interests to sit on advisory panels, it did not show similar generosity to a breast implant critic. The 1992 FDA advisory panel on silicone breast implant safety included one Baltimore doctor, Norman Anderson, whose voting privilege on that panel was canceled by the FDA, who claimed he was biased. According to a February 13, 1992, Associated Press release, Anderson had been influential in getting the FDA to reinvestigate breast implant safety and had publicly advocated removal of implants from the market. The FDA explained that Anderson's statements to media "led to an appearance of his inability to render objective advice."

Eli Lilly Provides Professional Services at APA

Eli Lilly is a powerful American corporation, but Prozac, with its 1993 sales of $1 billion, has given it a special place in psychiatry and within America itself. In May 1992 at the American Psychiatric Association meetings, Lilly's display in the exhibition hall was by far the largest, eighteen-by-thirty-six paces, the size and quality of a well-appointed hotel lobby. *Washington Post* reporter Joel Achenbach interviewed me on site as I gave him a tour of the fabulous displays aimed at turning on America's psychiatrists to even higher rates of drug prescription. He quoted me describing the annual psychiatric meeting as "the World's Fair of drug companies." Virtually the entire giant meeting was bought and paid for by the drug companies—everything from "scientific panels" to the message center and the lavish entertainment. Organized psychiatry couldn't run its conventions or scientific meetings, its newspapers or its journals, its media outreach programs or its lobbying office, without drug company money.[22]

Lilly Provides a "Service" to Practicing Physicians

Drug company advertisements are supposed to meet stringent standards for truthfulness and educational value set down by the FDA, but it is widely acknowledged that the FDA has neither the manpower nor the will to monitor the profusion of ads in medical journals. A 1992 survey by the Office of the Inspector General of the Department of Health and Human Services, for example, found that the majority of ads failed to meet medical or FDA standards. The investigation found that many ads lack educational value and that many are misleading and unscientific, with false claims for special advantages.

Meanwhile, according to the Inspector General's Office, as of 1990 the FDA "had not successfully prosecuted a violative drug advertiser in 23 years," but had begun to do so in 1991.

In this light, consider a multicolor ad for Prozac in the January 1994 issue of *The Journal of Clinical Psychiatry*. Dominated by the picture of a troubled face, it offers only a five-word headline and a short checklist. The complete headline reads "First line for all nine . . ." And below the picture, there is a checklist of nine "symptoms of depression," directly implying that Prozac should be the first choice in regard to each of them. The symptoms are "depressed mood, sleep disturbances, slowness/restlessness, loss of interest, weight/appetite change, guilt/feelings of worthlessness, fatigue, lack of concentration, thoughts of death."*

In what possible sense is Prozac "first line" for all of these symptoms? In terms of efficacy, Prozac is no better than many other antidepressants and, in the FDA trials, was usually less effective than the old-time tricyclics. Furthermore, Prozac is a poor and even hazardous choice for many of the nine symptoms. It is dangerous to give Prozac to depressed people who suffer from the most common form of "sleep disturbance," insomnia. It can drastically worsen the insomnia, potentially driving the patient into desperation. Prozac is similarly a poor choice for depressed patients who undergo the most frequent type of weight and appetite problem, loss of appetite. As Richard Kapit's in-house FDA evaluation suggested, Prozac can make people seem or feel more depressed by inducing greater weight loss and insomnia (see chapter 4). Similarly, in patients suffering from "restlessness," Prozac runs the risk of producing akathisia, agitation, or mania, with severe behavioral abnormalities, including violence against self or others. Prozac can also worsen loss of interest, lack of concentration, and especially thoughts of death.

Notice that last item—Prozac being promoted as "first line" for treating thoughts of death. Seriously suicidal people were excluded from the FDA trials, and the drug has been implicated as a cause of obsessive, violent suicidal thoughts.

Lilly's Prozac ad could lead physicians into dangerous prescribing practices with very harmful consequences. It has been known for some time that a large portion of physicians, however much they deny it, tend to be greatly influenced by drug company advertising and salespersons

---

*As required by law, the next page of the journal contains, in fine print, a portion of the drug's label. All journal ads do meet that formal requirement.

("detail men"). A 1982 study by Jerry Avorn and colleagues from Harvard Medical School found that commercial rather than scientific sources of information sway doctors and tend to miseducate them. The Harvard group's prime example was another Lilly product, Darvon, whose efficacy was overestimated by half the doctors surveyed.

Lilly Offers "Public Service" Through the National Mental Health Association

On March 10, 1994, we received an information packet we had requested from the National Mental Health Association via their 800 number. In addition to a slip of paper asking for memberships or donations, the packet contained two items. One was a pamphlet entitled "Answers to Your Questions About Clinical Depression." It provides a checklist to test yourself for depression and talks about how people are relieved to learn that depression is a "medical illness" and that "medical research has produced a variety of effective new medications to treat the illness." At the back of the brochure is the Eli Lilly logo and a statement: "Provided as a public service through an educational grant from Eli Lilly and Company." The other item in the envelope is a photocopy of the March 26, 1990, *Newsweek* cover story with a giant headline, "PROZAC: A Breakthrough Drug for Depression," and a picture of the honored Pulvule itself.

Why would the National Mental Health Association go so far out of its way to promote Lilly and Prozac? Because Lilly had infused the ailing philanthropic organization with an estimated $3 to $4 million for a national campaign on depression.[23] In addition to the massive campaign, individual state mental health associations would each be given $5,000. In return, they spewed a tidal wave of Lilly promotional materials across the nation.

The *Wall Street Journal*, which usually lavishes its support on the drug companies, raised questions in its head-line, "Critics See Self-Interest in Lilly's Funding of Ads Telling the Depressed to Get Help."[24] The newspaper observed, "The campaign is the most recent twist in a controversial trend in which pharmaceutical companies use consumer advertising to drive sales of prescription drugs."

An April 10, 1994, *New York Times* column by Elisabeth Rosenthal observed, "Some psychiatrists were infuriated by last year's multimedia advertising campaign sponsored by the National Mental Health Association." Drug companies argue that these campaigns are educational but, according to Rosenthal, many physicians disagree. She cites Marcus Reidenberg, M.D., editor of the *Journal of Clinical Pharmacology and Therapeutics*, as stating that drug companies "are taking symptoms of daily living, of normal existence, and converting these into diseases requiring medical treatment."

Rosenthal also quotes David A. Kessler, M.D., the Commissioner of the FDA, concerning consumer-oriented drug company campaigns in general. Kessler believes that "The effort is directed at getting people to walk into their doctor and demand a pill." Kessler also said of the drug companies, "They're not educating people about the medicines they take—which is what needs to be done—they're trying to increase demand."

Lilly Offers "Public Service" Through the National Institute of Mental Health

Before we come down too hard on the National Mental Health Association, it should be noted that Lilly had already established a similar hand-in-glove relationship with the National Institute of Mental Health and other federal agencies. In the 1980s, the NIMH developed a massive PR program for biopsychiatry called "D/ART—DE-PRESSION/Awareness, Recognition, Treatment," aimed at encouraging more people to see psychiatrists and especially to take drugs.[25] Among its many projects, D/ART produced a pamphlet, "Depression: What You Need to Know," that included special mention of serotonergic drugs. At that time, Lilly's Prozac was the only one available. Lilly supported the publication of the project, which has received mass distribution with Lilly and the government sharing credit for it. A statement says, "Printed and distributed as a public service" by the drug company.

In his "Beat the Devil" column in *The Nation* (January 31, 1994), Alexander Cockburn takes Lilly and NIMH's director, Frederick Goodwin,* to task for collaborating in trying to convince massive numbers of Americans that they suffer from depression. The government report and press conference were supported by Eli Lilly. Warns Cockburn, "Even now N.I.M.H.–type zealots may be brooding how to get Prozac into the national synapses, inhibiting serotonin re-uptake, getting people on the even, zombielike keel foreseen by Aldous Huxley with soma in *Brave New World*." Another public service from Eli Lilly.

Eli Lilly Provides "Public Service" Through the Government

Can Lilly and other drug companies directly influence government agencies? The Foundation for Advanced Education in the Sciences (FAES)[26] is a private foundation whose membership consists of National Institutes of Health (NIH) employees and "alumni." Until very recently, it for many years funneled millions of dollars to NIH scientists. The donations came from a variety of sources, including pharmaceutical companies. The first accounting we received included grants from Pfizer, A.H. Robins, G.D. Searle, CIBA-Geigy, Merrell Dow, Sandoz, Upjohn, Hoffman-La Roche, Abbott Labs, Du Pont, Bristol-Myers, and Eli Lilly, among others.

*Recently resigned.

The pharmaceutical firms used FAES to specify to whom their money would be donated and for what purposes. Through the Freedom of Information Act, we found, for example, that biopsychiatrist Judith L. Rapoport, chief of NIMH's Child Psychiatry Branch and a key person in pushing the use of drugs on children, has been receiving money from Eli Lilly and from CIBA-Geigy, the makers of Ritalin.[27] The CIBA-Geigy money was specified for research trying to demonstrate that childhood disorders are biological in nature—and hence, suitable for drug treatment.

Recent concerns about potential conflicts of interest have now caused the government to require that drug companies give the money directly to the federal agencies without strings attached concerning its use. FAES had to turn over $4 million in gifts to be administered by NIH. Since then, the drug companies have severely cut back on this aspect of their "public service," plunging FAES into financial difficulty.[28]

Meanwhile, Lilly finds other ways to influence government. According to a *New York Times* story by Neil Lewis, Lilly ranks third among drug companies in donations to members of Congress.

Lilly Buys a "Public Servant"

Psychiatrist Steven M. Paul was still scientific director of NIMH in March 1993 when he wrote an Op Ed feature for the *Wall Street Journal*. Announcing that he was moving on to become a vice-president of Eli Lilly, Paul defended drug companies against the criticism about excess profits and high prices being directed at them by President Clinton.

Lilly's hiring of one of the most influential men in government mental health research smacks of the military-industrial complex. As long as this can take place, federal researchers and administrators are bound to be motivated to seek favor with the giant drug companies. It can end up guaranteeing a lot more than a government pension. We don't think it's "public service" that led Paul to defend drug company products.[29]

We don't think it's chance that, in the last few years, federal health researchers have been vigorously supporting the possibility that drugs like Prozac might be used for the control of potential violence on a wide scale in America. In doing so, the government is trying to open up the greatest possible market ever envisioned for a drug violence—prevention and control. Toward this end, the government has been paying for research aimed at showing that violence is genetic, that it can be caused by serotonergic imbalances, and that SSRIs may be able to cure it.*

Lilly Offers "Public Service" Through President Bush and Vice-President Quayle

Corporations in general have had increasing influence over government policy under the Reagan–Bush administrations, but especially close ties existed between Eli Lilly and both Bush and Quayle. Before he ran for vice-president, George Bush was on the Board of Directors of Lilly, and as vice-president he continued to lobby on behalf of the company's interests.[30] Before his financial holdings were placed in a blind trust, Bush owned $90,000 of Lilly stock.

According to the *National Journal*, as vice-president Bush "repeatedly intervened to help the [drug] industry," for example, by easing the first stage of the FDA approval process for drugs in general.[31] Could these eased regulations have contributed to the recent deaths from liver failure in association with an Eli Lilly anti-hepatitis drug as

*We review this research in our forthcoming book, *The War Against Children*, to be published by St. Martin's Press this fall (1994).

it was undergoing early stages of testing at NIH? Sidney Wolfe, M.D., Director of Nader's health research group, has accused Lilly of failing to make required reports to the FDA concerning the hazards of this drug in time to save later experimental subjects from fatal side effects. Lilly denies any negligence. The law requires reporting only if it is known that the complications were directly related to the drug. Researchers did not attribute the liver failures to the hepatitis drug.*[32]

Coming from Indiana, Eli Lilly's home state, Dan Quayle naturally had close ties to the corporation, which supported him in his senatorial campaign. *The Nation* reports that as head of the Council on Competitiveness, Quayle asked Lilly to help reevaluate the FDA approval process to make it more to the liking of industry.[33] Undoubtedly Lilly's contribution was seen as one more public service.

According to a 1992 report by Ransdell Pierson in the *New York Post*, Quayle did succeed in cutting several years off the time most drugs require for FDA approval. More important, perhaps, the coalition between Quayle and Lilly surely must have been known to FDA officials during the Prozac approval process.[34]

Could these ties have influenced the FDA's rush to approve Prozac despite its demonstrated lack of efficacy and dangerous stimulant profile? Bureaucratic administrators are exquisitely responsive to pressures, direct or indirect, from the White House and Executive Office Building, and

*This is not the first time Lilly has been accused of negligence in connection with its drug testing. According to a 1985 *New York Times* story by Philip Shenon, the company pleaded guilty to "criminal charges that it failed to inform the Federal Government about four deaths and six illnesses related to its arthritis drug Oraflex." More recently, Lilly's factories have also drawn criticism. Without any mention of actual harm to patients, a 1993 *Wall Street Journal* story by Thomas Burton reported that one of the company's plants that makes emergency defibrillators had been closed down in response to an FDA investigation. Problems were also being investigated at other Lilly manufacturing facilities.

the mere knowledge of the Bush and Quayle ties to Lilly could have made them overly sensitive to the interests of the drug company.

The FDA, L-Tryptophan, and Drug Industry Profits

In 1989 the ingestion of the food supplement L-tryptophan was associated with more than 1,500 cases of a rare and potentially fatal disease, Eosinophilia-Myalgia Syndrome (EMS). An amino acid, L-tryptophan is used by the brain to manufacture serotonin. Since the late 1960s it's been used as a relatively safe, inexpensive, non-prescription alternative to psychiatric drugs for such disorders as insomnia, depression, and anxiety.

When Lilly and other drug companies began promoting their expensive, dangerous serotonergic agents, millions of people had already been using L-tryptophan for many years. But following the outbreak of EMS, L-tryptophan was taken off the market and then banned by the FDA in March 1992. Even though the problem was eventually traced to a specific contaminated batch of L-tryptophan produced in Japan, all L-tryptophan remains banned.[35]

Those who look critically at the FDA and the psycho-pharmaceutical complex have voiced concerns that the continuation of the L-tryptophan ban will force people to use SSRIs instead.

Lilly Provides "Public Service" Through the American Justice System

In chapter 5 we described the case of Dwight Harlor III, in which I participated as an expert witness and took the position that Prozac had played a role in producing his violence against his former wife. After it became clear that Harlor was using a "Prozac defense," Eli Lilly contacted the prosecution and offered to help them undermine my testimony and to build their case against Dwight. Dwight Harlor wasn't going up just against the state prosecutor, he was going up against one of the wealthiest and most savvy corporations in the nation.

After the case was over, I spoke by telephone with the assistant prosecuting attorney, Dennis Hogan, who was in charge of the case, and asked him if Lilly had offered any financial help. Hogan immediately responded, "I told them it would be unethical for the prosecution to accept funding." But on further questioning, he could not recall exactly what kind of financial help they had volunteered. He did remember that Lilly provided him the names of expert witnesses, background information on the issue of Prozac and violence, research studies, and a long list of questions to ask me on cross-examination. It was apparent to me that Hogan didn't want to fill me in on the details.

According to Dwight's attorney, Ed Davila of Canton, Ohio, Lilly also provided Hogan with a large tabulated document, about one and one-half inches thick, including a biography of me and statements I have made in print and to the media. Lilly also provided transcripts and summaries from a previous Prozac defense trial in which Davila was involved. In addition, it offered free, unlimited assistance from a major Columbus, Ohio, law firm to help with research, advice, and related activities. The long list of questions to ask me on cross-examination would have taken a day to answer. According to Davila, he and Hogan laughed about how most of the questions were irrelevant to Dwight's case, but seemingly of interest to Lilly for other purposes or occasions.

According to Davila, Assistant Prosecutor Hogan told him that Lilly also offered to fund the prosecution's expenses, including the high cost of experts. Davila explained to me that Hogan, a former public defender, rejected the financial offers as unethical, but made use of the huge store of information sent to him.

Davila explained that Lilly had made similar overtures of financial assistance to the state prosecutor in an earlier

Prozac defense case he was defending. In that instance, the prosecutor had confirmed in court that Lilly offered to fund the state's case and that the state had, in that instance as well, rejected the funding as unethical.

The Harlor case was a defeat for Eli Lilly in that the Prozac defense contributed to his staying out of jail. But Davila believes that Lilly probably prefers these negotiated plea bargains to court battles, since they contribute to a false conclusion that no Prozac defense cases have come out successfully.

Lilly's involvement in the Harlor case is part of an overall company strategy. Lilly has been intervening vigorously in the criminal justice system on behalf of state prosecutors in order to discredit the "Prozac defense."[36] Lilly doesn't want the courts putting their imprimatur on the idea that Prozac can cause violent and criminal behavior and so, in effect, it gangs up on ordinary citizens who lack the financial clout to fight off both the state and one of the nation's most powerful corporations.

According to Amy Marcus in the *Wall Street Journal*, an attorney remarked on the Lilly strategy:

> Not only am I fighting the prosecutor, now I'm fighting the resources of Eli Lilly. That isn't fair when I'm trying to defend someone [who is] on a limited budget in a capital case.

Another observed:

> Permitting a multibillion-dollar private enterprise to join in a consortium with a government prosecutorial agency raises very strong constitutional issues relating to a defendant's right to a fair trial.

In order to discourage malpractice suits against doctors who prescribe Prozac, Lilly has guaranteed to fund the defense of any physician who prescribes Prozac according to accepted practice.[37] Since dozens of malpractice suits have been brought against physicians who prescribe Prozac, this is a big promise, aimed once again at keeping Prozac's image untarnished. Lilly made the offer at a moment when it looked as if sales might be hurt by accusations that its antidepressant could cause suicide and murder.[38]

Many drug companies vie with Lilly for influence in the psycho-pharmaceutical complex.[39] Lilly has merely taken center stage with the success of Prozac. Now that Bush and Quayle are out of office, perhaps Congress could begin an investigation of drug company influence in America, perhaps starting with Lilly's intervention in the justice system.

We have discussed the story of Margaret McCaffrey, whose daughter, a neurologist, killed herself while taking Prozac. On November 8, 1993, Congressman Edolphus Towns, chairman of the House Subcommittee on Human Resources and Intergovernmental Relations, wrote to Prozac survivor Margaret McCaffrey to explain that he is planning a future investigation of the FDA's approval process for psychiatric drugs, including Prozac. The public should remind Congressman Towns to make this a top priority.

NINE

How and Why to Stop Taking Psychiatric Drugs

Nowadays it is fashionable, although unproven, to think of depression as genetic and biochemical in origin, and to turn to drugs as the answer. We have seen that many professional and economic interests drive society in this direction.* We now turn to some of the more personal motivations that people have for relying on psychiatric drugs, and we introduce the basic principles of how to withdraw from these medications.

DEPRESSION OFTEN SEEMS TO BE PHYSICAL

Depression often has a physical feeling to it. It's as if the brain has become gummed up, the body slowed down. The person has trouble focusing attention or recalling simple things, and may worry that these symptoms herald the onset of Alzheimer's disease or a brain tumor. Weight loss is common, although weight gain occurs as well. Insomnia is frequent. Sometimes, instead of feeling sluggish, the depressed person feels driven or agitated, as if trying to escape the unseen, unnamed enemy; and again, the inner pressure can easily feel physical in origin.

*Also see Breggin, *Toxic Psychiatry*, 1991, chapter 15, Psychiatry and the Psycho-Pharmaceutical Complex.

In the extreme, the afflicted individual begins to harbor fantasies that reach a delusional scale—bodily organs deteriorating, an awful smell emanating from one's pores, worms crawling out of the skin. Spiritual torment becomes transformed into physical sensations and fantasies, and other unreal imaginings.

Because depression often is associated with physical symptoms, people are prone to view it as biological in origin. But the presence of physical symptoms by no means suggests a physical cause. Fear of being mugged, for example, can cause the heart to beat faster, the pupils to enlarge, the hands to tremble, the blood pressure to rise, and the skin to sweat. Similarly, great joy at greeting a loved one can take our breath away, bring color to our faces, cause us to tremble, and sometimes bring tears to our eyes. In neither case should the physical response be used as evidence for a physical cause.

Our dog, Blue, gets dreadfully depressed when we leave him overnight at the veterinarian, where he languishes in a tiny cage side by side with other desperate and lonely animals. He stops eating and loses weight. After a recent overnight at the vet's, he "blew his coat"—huge gobs of his magnificent fur fell out. These are physical symptoms from an emotional distress.

People also come to believe that depression is physical because it's so painful, so overwhelming, so extreme. They feel as if they are "sick" and they often look ill. But that's the way human emotions affect us. Children and primates who are emotionally abandoned can fail to thrive and even die. Their anguish is psychological in origin, but it becomes lethal to their physical body. That desperation, despair, or other emotional responses have become extreme does not prove that they have a biological or genetic origin.

Emotional stress can produce physical changes in the body. Steroid and adrenaline production, for example, can markedly increase, and the output of sexual hormones can decrease. Severe inner conflict and stress can cause or worsen physical diseases, including a number that afflict the cardiovascular and digestive systems, and the skin and hair. But the development of these physical symptoms takes place without an underlying genetic or biological cause.

The idea of having a "disease" can be appealing when we lack confidence in our capacity to overcome our problems. If depression is a disease, then we take encouragement from turning to doctors. And we can stop blaming ourselves so much. All this is very understandable and very human, but it's not necessarily the correct or best way to view human suffering and its relief.

Being human, having suffered in our own lives, and having shared the suffering of those near and dear to us, we can easily understand the temptation to fall back on "I have a disease." But experience has taught us that it's best at all times to stay in charge of our own lives—to understand, to grow, to seek meaningful comforts, and to empower ourselves, however difficult it may seem at any given moment.

HOW PSYCHIATRISTS OFTEN TAKE ADVANTAGE

Frightened, helpless-feeling, self-blaming people can easily be influenced by authorities who promise them relief and absolution, which is what many psychiatrists do when they claim that depression is genetic and biological in origin and can be relieved with a pill. In a sense, psychiatrists take advantage of the patients' worst feelings about themselves. Patients seek professional advice because they feel helpless and personally defective. The psychiatrist says, in effect, "You are helpless and defective, but it's a physical disease rather than a mental or moral failing." Depression, in reality, is neither a disease nor a moral failing. It is a psychological signal that an individual has become stymied and overwhelmed and needs to find a new approach to life.

Psychiatrists have been claiming that depression is physical or biological ever since the inception of the profession hundreds of years ago. Despite all the media coverage about this "new" understanding of depression, it's a very old theme. Why have so many psychiatrists continually claimed that depression is biological? The answer is simple: Because they are physicians. As physicians, they are trained to examine problems at the physiological level. As physicians, they are trained to treat physical diseases. If they concluded that human suffering was psychological and spiritual rather than medical in origin, psychiatrists would have to give up trying to help depressed people through medicine. Some psychiatrists are willing to do this, but they are the exception. For most psychiatrists, their training, professional identity, authority, standing in the community, and income are tied up with the validity of the medical approach.

Meanwhile, there is no substantial scientific evidence that depression is physical or genetic. While this conclusion may be stunning to the reader who is familiar with the psychiatric propaganda that graces the science sections of newspapers and magazines, it is scientifically incontrovertible. While some physical diseases, such as thyroid disorders or Cushing's disease, are sometimes associated with depressed feelings, there is no convincing evidence that any problem routinely seen by psychiatrists has a genetic or biological origin.*

THE LESSONS OF ALCOHOL FOR PROZAC USERS

While profoundly distressed people sometimes feel relief and encouragement when told they have a genetic and biological disease, there are other more unfortunate ef-

---

*A critical examination of the various genetic and biological theories can be found in my books *Toxic Psychiatry* and *The War Against Children*, co-written with Ginger Ross Breggin.

fects that I often discover in my practice. Convinced that they have a genetic-biochemical defect, depressed people can end up believing that they are stuck forever with being "ill." These false biological principles can become frightening to anyone struggling with a bout of depression. Families begin to remember that Aunt Harriet or Grandfather Paul was probably depressed, and fears are magnified for the currently depressed family member. Everyone aligns with the psychiatrist in trying to convince the family member to take drugs for the duration of his or her life in order to manage the otherwise inexorable disease. In clinical practice, this is becoming an increasing problem, as therapeutic efforts run counter to the patient's conviction, gleaned from the media, that he or she has a biochemical imbalance.

Biochemical and genetic theories leave patients feeling dependent on experts. Sometimes they go from doctor to doctor hoping someone will come up with the right medical diagnosis or drug treatment. If they remain depressed, a biologically oriented psychiatrist will eventually recommend electroshock, a treatment more likely to permanently wreck than to improve a life.[1]

In my view, patients who become enmeshed in biopsychiatry often become victimized by what I have called "iatrogenic* denial in authoritarian psychiatry."[2] Any drug—including alcohol—that affects the mind is actually producing brain dysfunction. This diminishes the victim's capacity for self-insight, especially in regard to the degree of dysfunction he or she is experiencing. Some of this denial is physiological in origin and some is a psychological defense against dealing with impairment.

Our knowledge of the effects of alcohol provides a valuable lesson for Prozac users. If you are taking any kind of psychoactive drug, from Prozac to cocaine or alcohol, it's important to realize that the drug itself can drastically

*Doctor- or treatment-caused.

compromise your ability to assess its impact on your mind and body.

In recent years the ads have said: "Friends don't let friends drive drunk." But have you ever tried to take away a drunk friend's car keys? Your friend is certain he can drive circles around you, at the very moment that he's barely able to rise from his barstool. This is very important for anyone reading this book: You may, or may not, be in a position to judge the true effect that any drug, including Prozac, is having on your mind.

People who have thought that alcohol helps them socialize are sometimes appalled when they give up drinking and go sober to the same parties. They realize they were fooling themselves all along. They weren't socializing in any real sense. They were being drunk with a lot of other drunks. All of a sudden, what once seemed like superior performance now appears like a disability.

If you yourself are taking Prozac, remember the lesson from alcohol: The person taking a psychoactive drug is impaired in his or her ability to judge its effect. You may feel better than ever—but you may not be. Patients on Prozac may no longer perceive either the drug-induced toxicity or their personal problems. They may believe they are better off when, in reality, they are worse off. Meanwhile, the psychiatrist too often joins the patients in mutual iatrogenic denial by claiming that the treatment is harmless to the brain, that it produces no serious side effects, and that the patients have biochemical imbalances rather than emotional problems.

Patients who are prescribed drugs frequently tend to give up trying to understand themselves, including the sources of their problems and their potential for psychological or spiritual growth. They can become skeptical and despairing about the possibilities of overcoming depression through self-insight, improved principles of living, a better family life, a more inspiring occupation, and all of the other transformations that often lead to spiritual triumph.

With increasing frequency, psychiatrists tend to tell patients that their problems are not only biochemical but genetic. When people are told that their emotional difficulties are genetic, they begin to look differently upon themselves. They can feel less able to personally deal with their problems. They may also change their attitudes toward their own children, who now seem vulnerable to the same or related genetic diseases. Instead of accepting the inevitable anguish of growing up, it becomes easy for these parents to see every difficulty as a sign of erupting disease in their children. Instead of examining and resolving conflicts within the family, or otherwise improving the child's home or school environment, they find professionals to help them blame everything on the youngster's genetic makeup. As a result, millions of children and adolescents end up on psychiatric drugs[3] or, as Louise Armstrong has described in *And They Call It Help*, they are thrown into mental hospitals.

ARE MY FEELINGS REAL OR JUST A DRUG SIDE EFFECT?

When depressed patients receive psychiatric drugs, the enormously confusing factor of toxicity is added to their emotional problems. Once a course of medication treatment for depression is begun, it becomes difficult to differentiate between adverse drug effects and the original depression, as well as other feelings, such as anxiety or anger. Patients on drugs have grave difficulty evaluating their mental condition, let alone the specific contribution of drugs to their upset. To add to their confusion, they have usually been told that the drugs are relatively harmless. In discussions among the committee members and consultants at the FDA Prozac hearing, for example, it was remarked that doctors often fail to tell Prozac patients about the most widely recognized side effects, such as insomnia or agitation, let alone the more controversial ones, like violence and suicide.

Patients and their families are rarely made aware that, when medication is stopped, withdrawal effects can mimic emotional problems. For the patient and family, it seems as if the illness is returning or some new emotional problem is surfacing.

Psychiatrists and other physicians commonly fail to distinguish between adverse drug effects and the individual's original depressed condition. Doctors encourage this confusion by talking about how drugs can "bring out underlying emotional problems" when, in fact, the drugs are *creating* them. Biased psychiatrists tend to attribute new symptoms to the patient's condition without exploring the possible need to reduce or stop the medication.

In chapter 7, for example, we saw how the most obvious twitches and spasms from neuroleptic-induced tardive dyskinesia have been blamed on "mental illness." Instead of withdrawing the neuroleptics and discovering the presence of a permanent neurological disease, the tendency was to increase the dose of the offending drug.* As a result, it took decades for the profession to recognize tardive dyskinesia, and, even today, it frequently goes unrecognized in actual practice.[4]

In the case of SSRIs, drug-induced agitation is likely to be treated with sedatives, which in themselves can cause agitation, creating a vicious cycle. Or drug-induced insomnia may be treated with sleep medications, which in themselves eventually become ineffective or produce rebound insomnia.[5] Or drug-induced depression, sometimes associated with withdrawal, will be treated with increased doses of the offending drug.

Many psychiatrists claim that they rarely if ever encounter serious withdrawal effects from antidepressants

---

*Increasing the dose of neuroleptics tends to temporarily suppress the symptoms while further damaging the brain and worsening the drug-induced neurological disease.

or, for that matter, from any psychiatric drugs. Yet I frequently deal with withdrawal reactions in my practice. Why is there this seeming difference in experience? In addition to the bias that keeps too many psychiatrists from confronting the harm that drugs can do, there is another factor.

When I realize the patient has developed significant new symptoms while on a drug, my tendency is to withdraw the medication, leading to the discovery that the symptoms then disappear. Also, I am frequently consulted by patients who feel unable to stop taking psychiatric drugs. In the treatment process, the patient and I often discover that stopping the medications brings about serious withdrawal symptoms.

In contrast, other psychiatrists tend to assume that any new symptoms are due to changes in the patient's emotional "pathology" rather than to drug effects. So they either increase the drug dose or prescribe an additional one. After a while, patients end up taking several drugs at once, and typically have more problems from unrecognized toxicity than from their original emotional problems.

FINDING HELP IN COMING OFF PSYCHIATRIC DRUGS

As the warning in the front of the book states, it can be very dangerous to withdraw from almost any psychiatric drug, and professional consultation and supervision is necessary.

If an individual is trying to withdraw from sedative or tranquilizing psychiatric drugs, such as Xanax or Valium, help is often available in the form of "detox centers" or other drug abuse programs. Almost every city has resources of this kind and local physicians or medical societies know how to locate them. On occasion, drug abuse facilities may be willing to accept a patient who is having trouble withdrawing from supposedly nonaddictive drugs, such as neuroleptics and antidepressants, but usually they will not.

Unfortunately, many psychiatrists have little experience withdrawing patients from antidepressant and neuroleptic drugs, and some display a limited inclination to learn more about it. Other than my own books and workshops, I don't know of any professionals who devote much time to this critical subject.

For individuals who are having trouble finding a psychiatrist who is sympathetic to withdrawal from supposedly nonaddictive psychiatric drugs, another approach is to locate an internist or general practitioner who will supervise the medical side of it. The patient can, at the same time, seek psychotherapeutic support from a nonmedical therapist, such as a clinical psychologist or social worker (see Appendix for information on how to locate a psychotherapist). Sometimes Twelve-Step programs can be helpful as well. Psychiatric survivor groups can also provide moral support and sometimes can direct people to sympathetic professionals (see Appendix for a listing of these groups).

UNDERSTANDING DRUG-WITHDRAWAL SYMPTOMS

Here are a few principles that can help professionals and consumers alike become more alert to drug-withdrawal problems:

1. *Any physical or emotional reaction that develops within a few hours or days after stopping a psychiatric drug may be due to withdrawal.*

   It may also be caused by a potentially debilitating fear of doing without the drug. It usually takes longer than a few hours or days after stopping the drug for the patient's original emotional problems to return.

2. *Any emotional reaction that is accompanied by phys-*

ical symptoms during or shortly after drug treatment should raise suspicions of a drug reaction, either toxicity or withdrawal.

During withdrawal, many tricyclic antidepressants and neuroleptics, for example, produce a flu-like syndrome with headache, muscle and joint aches, chills, nausea or vomiting, loss of appetite, and diarrhea, as well as insomnia and emotional distress.

3. *Any symptom that is opposite to the drug effect may be due to withdrawal.*

The brain almost always tries to overcome or compensate for the impact of a drug. As a result, withdrawal from a medication that causes sedation and sleep is likely to produce agitation and insomnia. Conversely, withdrawal from a drug that produces stimulation or alertness, including SSRIs, is likely to produce fatigue and dullness.

4. *Drug withdrawal commonly occurs during drug treatment as the brain tries to overcome the drug effect.*

Patients taking sleeping pills or minor tranquilizers at a fixed daily dose can find themselves developing insomnia and agitation, while patients taking stimulant drugs like Prozac or amphetamines can find themselves becoming fatigued, exhausted, and in need of sleep.

Drug withdrawal that takes place during drug treatment frequently manifests itself at that time of day when the drug effect is wearing off. Although hard evidence is not yet available, this is likely to be more obvious with the use of short-acting drugs such as Paxil or Zoloft, rather than with Prozac. When the drug is active in the body for a briefer time, withdrawal symptoms can arise more quickly and with more impact. If the drug is taken in the morning, withdrawal symptoms may turn up in the evening, and vice versa.

As a very short-acting drug, the sleeping pill Halcion can produce several withdrawal reactions by the next afternoon or early evening before the next dose is taken. Patients have been known to become agitated, disturbed, depressed, and violent while taking Halcion, sometimes as drug withdrawal occurs during the next day.[6]

PRINCIPLES OF DRUG WITHDRAWAL

The following principles may help professionals and patients with the drug-withdrawal process:

1. *It is not safe or desirable to use this book as the sole basis for withdrawing from psychiatric drugs.*
   Drug withdrawal requires the supervision of a competent, experienced professional.
2. *Respect the patient's wishes and right to know.*
   Despite the virtual monopoly over media coverage achieved by leaders in biological psychiatry, there is a broad range of opinion about the usefulness of psychiatric drugs within the mental health field and among consumers. Individual opinions, including those of patients, should be respected. When patients come to me, for example, I do not urge them to stop taking drugs unless there is an unequivocal immediate threat posed by drug toxicity. Rather, I try to inform them of all the relevant information, including the existence of viewpoints contrary to mine.* A physician may hold a position that differs from that of his or her patient, but should nonetheless pay attention to the opinions and subjective perceptions of the pa-

---

*Information in favor of drugs is so readily available that we feel no necessity to present the pro-drug view in this book. The Appendix, however, lists several commonly used sources of drug information in psychiatry, many of them devoted to the biopsychiatric approach. The argument in favor of Prozac is presented most recently and completely in Fieve, 1994, as well as in Jonas and Schaumburg, 1991, and in Kramer, 1993.

tient, and recognize the patient's right to seek a doctor who is like-minded.

During the process of withdrawal, it is especially important to focus on the patient's subjective responses. When patients ask me, "How long will it take for me to get off this drug?" I usually emphasize that it will take as long as necessary from the patient's viewpoint.

3. *Withdrawal from certain drugs can be extremely dangerous.*

Abruptly stopping large doses of sedatives and minor tranquilizers, especially shorter-acting ones like Xanax or Halcion, can be life-threatening. Withdrawal from some drugs, including sedatives and anticonvulsants, can produce seizures.

4. *Unless a physician determines that the patient is undergoing a toxic drug reaction that requires rapid withdrawal, it is best to err on the side of withdrawing too slowly rather than too rapidly.*

How much time to take for withdrawal is a complicated question, depending on the drug, its combination with other drugs, and the patient's health and subjective feelings. It requires a competent professional evaluation to determine the safety parameters for length of withdrawal. In general, however, most psychiatrists tend to withdraw drugs too rapidly, and then to err once again in reinstating them without giving the patient a chance to get through the withdrawal phase.

5. *If a patient is taking several psychiatric drugs, it is usually best to stop one drug at a time.*

Removing one medication at a time makes it easier for the doctor and patient to assess what is happening during the withdrawal process. As a corollary, if a patient is taking several psychiatric medications at once, it becomes impossible to disentangle their overall impact on the brain and mind. In regard to psychoactive drugs, the fewer the better is a good rule.

6. *Friends, family, and, if possible, co-workers should be alerted to the problems the patient will face while undergoing drug withdrawal.*

   Withdrawal from almost any psychiatric drug can result in emotional turmoil. My own clinical observations and reports from the national Prozac Survivor Support Group indicate that withdrawal from SSRIs like Prozac, Zoloft, or Paxil can cause dangerous abnormal behaviors. The patient may not recognize these responses due to drug-induced mental dysfunction.

7. *Most people need a support network to help them through drug withdrawal.*

   Physicians and mental health professionals often need to work with the patient's family and social network, including the patient's minister or medical doctor, during and after the withdrawal process. This is especially true if the patient has been on neuroleptic drugs for many years, because withdrawal can cause severe emotional turmoil and even psychosis. Friends and family may find their tolerance and patience tested, and if they are not involved in a supportive fashion, the effort is likely to fail.

   Withdrawing someone from drugs can be an arduous task, and the individual clinician might not be able to handle more than a few patients at a time. Ideally, it would often be best to call upon the resources of a full-service clinic, but few are willing to help patients withdraw from psychiatric drugs (see Appendix). Twelve-Step programs and survivor support groups can be helpful, too (see Appendix).

After coming off years of psychiatric drugs, many former patients decide to have nothing more to do with mental health professionals. Often they feel hurt, betrayed, and embittered. Yet there are many "talking doctors," including some psychiatrists and many other nonmedical professionals, who do have a great deal to offer. People who suffer from depression can often be helped by caring professional interventions, as well as through many other paths of their own choosing. In the final chapter, we will look at some of the essential principles for overcoming depression.

TEN

Understanding and Overcoming Depression

When I worked in mental hospitals during my psychiatric training, I often treated the most extremely depressed patients, some who were not eating or taking fluids, others who were actively suicidal. Some seemed destined for shock treatment or commitment to the state mental hospital until I began to work with them. Unlike many other severely impaired patients, those who were depressed almost always responded to caring psychotherapeutic interventions, often involving both individual and family therapy.*

Often I would devote several hours a day to the patient and family during the first week or so of hospitalization, but in the long run it was much less expensive or time-consuming than lengthy hospitalizations and persistent disability. But nearly all my young colleagues would have been uncomfortable with such intensive therapeutic involvements; they felt more comfortable and had more faith in drugs and shock treatment. Nothing in their background or training prepared them to be that "involved" with other people, and nearly everything primed them for being distant and controlling.

---

*I describe several of these treatment experiences in *Toxic Psychiatry* and elaborate on them more fully in my novel, *The Crazy from the Sane*.

In my private psychiatric practice, of course, fewer of my patients are in such bad shape. Under special circumstances, I will sometimes accept patients who might otherwise be treated in a mental hospital. They and their families typically come to me looking for an alternative after sometimes devastating failures at the hands of biological psychiatrists and mental hospitals. These patients usually need a local support network of friends or family and frequent sessions early in the therapy. While the initial psychotherapeutic treatment may be intensive, it is a tiny fraction of the cost of hospitalization.

I have never started one of my depressed patients on an antidepressant. For more than twenty-five years, I have instead done my best to get involved, to care, to understand, and to work with family and friends when needed. Because depression is such an obviously psychological and spiritual condition—a state of despair and hopelessness—it has always seemed to me that the dedicated involvement of caring human beings is the key.

In extreme circumstances, when patients won't eat, I will eat with them. Almost anyone will let a caring therapist feed them, especially if the therapist is eating with them, and the opportunity can lead to profound insights and improvements. When patients have been acutely suicidal, I have made myself available every day and tried to see to it that they had regular companionship; but I have not involuntarily hospitalized or drugged them.*

On occasion, an extremely depressed patient has decided to start on drugs with another psychiatrist while see-

---

*While I don't provide a home service, it would be easy to do so for patients who were homebound with their depression. It would also be much less expensive than mental hospitalization. If psychotherapy were not controlled by the mental health monopoly, innovations like that would be more common. Without the artificial inflation of prices by the monopoly, psychotherapy would also cost much less and therefore be more available.

ing me for psychotherapy. But almost always, the drugs
have turned out to do more harm than good. Often these
patients end up asking me to take over the drug treatment
in order to help wean them off the medication. While I
won't start patients on antidepressants, I will prescribe
these drugs if someone is already taking them or is in the
process of withdrawal.

Organized psychiatry acts as if drugs are a necessity,
but when giving workshops around the country, I find that
innumerable mental health professionals act on similar
principles to my own. They love and care for their patients, share emotionally and spiritually with them within
the limits of ethical therapy, help them understand the
roots of their depression, and provide inspiration and better psychological principles for taking on life once again.
My workshops give these professionals further courage to
pursue what they have always believed and found to be
true.

In the meanwhile, keep in mind that there's no evidence that antidepressants are especially effective as
treatments. In chapter 3 we found that Prozac, for example, was approved by the FDA with studies that excluded hospitalized or seriously suicidal patients. In the
majority of FDA studies, Prozac proved equal to or only
a little better than a sugar pill but a lot more hazardous.
In not giving antidepressants, we are not depriving patients of a "miracle cure." We are instead giving them an
important message—that they have the psychological and
spiritual resources to triumph over depression and to
make a life that is better than they ever hoped for.

THE SUFFERING OF DEPRESSION IS REAL

The National Institute of Mental Health (NIMH), a federal agency that promotes the interests of organized psychiatry, has estimated that almost 10 million Americans
are seriously depressed and that a total of 14 million will

suffer from it during their lifetimes. In response to escalating estimates from the psychiatric establishment, some media have been citing figures of up to 20 million sufferers at any one time.

These estimates are presented to the public as factual data, but they are distributed to the media through carefully organized psychiatric promotional campaigns backed by national organizations, like the American Psychiatric Association and the National Institute of Mental Health, as well as private drug companies. They aim to encourage people to seek medical help for emotional problems.[1] While it is true that depression is a common and deeply distressing human problem, defining it as a biological disease requiring medical treatment is a sales campaign. The message means a lot of business for drug companies and psychiatry.

The choice of people instead of pills as a method of helping is in no way intended to minimize the suffering experienced during depression. Depression is one of the most dreadful human experiences. Too often, it ruins lives or leads to suicide, with a spread of effect that spoils the lives of others as well. Even people who do not seem depressed may be diluting their emotional pain with alcohol, drug abuse, or other self-destructive activities, such as participation in a degrading relationship or reckless behavior while driving an automobile. They may end up killing themselves or dying of self-neglect, without being recorded as a suicide.

The experience of depression is often felt as dark and cold—utterly bleak—as if subsisting in a cave or hole. Life loses its sunshine. Nothing seems enjoyable anymore. Eventually, depression can deteriorate into self-hate and loathing.

Some of the most frightening descriptions of depression have come from famous, successful people who have "come out of the closet." Often, they describe being unable to get out of bed, and feeling intensely suicidal. Hearing their stories moves us with pity. On a bad day or at a difficult time in our lives, we may recall their experiences and become fearful that their kind of depression has entered our own lives.

Many people go through life with what might be called a "low-grade" depression. They are apathetic and life seems monotonous with nothing to look forward to. There are no highs anymore, nothing to delight the senses, the heart, or the mind. Life may not seem utterly dark, but it's gray. Lacking in energy, seemingly unable to find any brightness in life, life becomes a treadmill of boredom and bleakness.

Some people have been depressed for so long that they hardly realize that their suffering is unusual. They become convinced that it's an inevitable response to life. Mired down in futility, they never change their lives.

DEPRESSION IS A COMMON HUMAN EXPERIENCE

Depression is such a common human experience that almost everyone has undergone some degree of it. Many people in the northeast, for example, get the "winter blues." In hot and humid climates, the onset of summer may produce the same effect. Others start to feel "down" with the approach of the holiday season. People often feel depressed when they get overtired or fatigued and cannot carry on with their usual energy. They can feel depressed if something much desired hasn't materialized, like a date or a promotion. Many grown men get a terrible sinking feeling that can last for days when their favorite sports team loses a championship game. The flu, exhaustion, mild head injury, and many transient physical stresses can be accompanied by depression. These feelings are usually temporary, but they give us a sense of what depression might be like if it were infinitely intensified and drawn out, as if one were never getting what one wanted . . . as if one were doomed always to lose.

More devastating feelings of depression are also surprisingly common. Probably most teenagers and young people go through moods of utter despair, often tinged with suicidal feelings, in their struggle to outgrow childhood and to find their identities. Probably most elderly people go through a similar struggle for a time at least as friends and family pass away or as they themselves approach death. The cycles of life include emotional cycles.

Almost anyone will go through severe feelings of depression with the loss of a loved one. Religions tend to recognize this inevitability and to provide for ritualized periods of mourning in which the bereaved are given special attention.

Research many years ago documented how infants and small children respond by withdrawing into depression when abandoned or rejected. More recently, a large body of research on physical, emotional, and sexual abuse in childhood confirms that it can contribute to lifelong depression.[2] These observations have been proven again and again by studies of individuals who go through cataclysmic stresses and losses, from concentration camps to wars. Clinicians like myself have seen this confirmed time and again. Usually when I get to know the life story of a client or new friend who seems depressed, I marvel that they have done as well as they have, considering what they've been through.

Animals, too, go through depression. Wild animals, for example, frequently become depressed when locked up in zoos. They refuse to mate and may languish and die. Pets frequently become depressed when their owners leave them behind for a day or more. They may stop eating and act mopey or resentful when the loved one returns. The owner may even find uncharacteristic destruction—a chewed shoe or emptied wastebasket—as a sign of the pet's frustration.

Jane Goodall in *Chimpanzees of Gombe* describes how infant chimps inevitably become depressed and die if they lose their mother within the first few years of life. Adolescent chimps who survive the loss may, at a somewhat later age, display emotional scars. They may be irritable and withdrawn, socially inept, and less able to take care of themselves or their own offspring as adults. In *Gorillas in the Mist*, Dian Fossey described similar responses in mountain gorillas.

Anyone who thinks that depression is caused by genetic and biochemical factors in humans ought to read these primate studies, which show depression's psychospiritual origins in "lower animals." Chimpanzees and gorillas are presumably more controlled by heredity and anatomy than human beings, yet their lives show them as extraordinarily sensitive to environmental stresses and remarkably responsive to loving interventions. These results have been confirmed again and again in primate studies in labs and natural habitats as well.

It's ironic that students of animal life now credit them with qualities previously reserved for humans, including the capacity for empathy, love, loss, and depression—at the very moment that psychiatrists have decided that humans are ruled by more animalistic forces of nature.

LOVE AND HOPE: THE NON-DRUG APPROACH TO OVERCOMING DEPRESSION

What alternatives are available for people who feel depressed?

Depression is a human—or animal—response to painful life circumstances, frequently in the form of losses. Everyone's personal experiences, as well as clinical and experimental research, confirm this. Depression lifts whenever a person regains hope and direction. Everyone has seen this happen, if not in oneself, then in other people.

We mentioned earlier how our dog, Blue, becomes depressed when caged overnight at the vet's. But he does fine when he stays at the kennel. Why? At the kennel, our friends Tom and Gerry let him romp all day with the other dogs in the large yard and at night he comes in to sit beside Tom on the couch in front of the television. Blue is a favorite of Tom's and favorites don't usually get depressed, unless there's a price attached to the favoritism.

So even Blue, a somewhat simple creature, doesn't need pills to ward off depression. The cure isn't a drug; it's being with people who love him.

Just as seemingly trivial stresses or losses can vault some people into depression, so too almost any hope can lift them from it. We have already noted that a large percentage of seriously depressed patients in double-blind placebo-controlled experiments will feel improved as a result of getting a sugar pill.*

Depression is especially responsive to changes in circumstances and relationships. A fan in the stands during a championship game may cycle through despair and euphoria as the tide turns one way and then another. Similarly, people go up and down emotionally through the experiences of their intimate relationships. Often depression is lifted by falling in love, making a new friend, adopting a pet, learning a new skill, joining a church, traveling, participating in volunteer or reform work, throwing oneself into work, or simply through the passage of time. Sometimes depression is relieved when an oppressive spouse or parent dies; or sometimes, due to guilt, it becomes worse. Time by itself—and probably the personal resources and new experiences that surface as time passes—seems to cure the vast majority of depressions.

*The problem has so embarrassed and confounded drug research that frequently a "placebo washout" is employed to identify and exclude from continuation in the controlled study those people who respond to the mere anticipation of getting help from a new medication (see chapter 3).

THERAPY AS A TREATMENT FOR DEPRESSION

The depressed person lacks hope and usually suffers from dreadful, self-punishing, self-blaming ideas. If the therapist can inspire hope and, at the same time, help dissipate the feelings of guilt—the worst aspects of severe depressions can often be speedily overcome through psychotherapy. This is much more true for depression than for a whole variety of other difficulties, especially those where the individual tends to blame someone else as the source of the problem, or where the feelings of emotional pain are locked inside obsessions and compulsions, or suppressed by addictions.

Scientific studies comparing psychotherapy to medication are not very useful. Good therapists are hard to find, and a person needs to shop around for someone with whom there is good rapport. This doesn't happen during research projects. Good therapists are usually eclectic, using a variety of approaches depending upon the individual's needs, while research projects tend to compare one carefully circumscribed form of therapy, for example, cognitive therapy, to drug therapy. Psychotherapy usually requires time, and patients like to know the time is available, while research projects usually end after a few weeks. Finally, research projects are usually skewed to drugs by emphasizing symptom relief, such as weight gain or improved sleep, which can easily be affected by drugs. More important variables are usually omitted, such as improved quality of inner life, higher hopes for the future, or new and more adventuresome behavior. Even so, as we described in chapter 3, these studies often fail to demonstrate a positive drug effect.

Even though most research is conducted by investigators with a strong bias toward drugs, psychiatric propaganda about the superiority of drugs over psychotherapy is wholly misleading. In terms of how patients actually feel and view life after treatment, psychotherapy is superior to drugs. A good review can be found in Seymour Fisher and Roger Greenberg's 1989 book, *The Limits of Biological Treatments for Psychological Distress: Comparisons with Psychotherapy and Placebo.*

In August 1993 I was on a panel at the annual convention of the American Psychological Association in Toronto, Canada, with David Antonuccio, Ph.D., a psychologist and associate professor at the University of Nevada School of Medicine and V.A. Medical Center in Reno. He reviewed those studies that claim superiority for drugs over psychotherapy in depression and found that the studies themselves often showed that psychotherapy worked better. Antonuccio declared:

> In conclusion, we feel that clinicians need to learn to resist the urge to deliver the quick fix in the form of a pill despite considerable pressure from the medical establishment, the media, and even the patient to do so. One cannot heal the soul with a medication. We tend to overlook the power of a caring psychotherapeutic relationship in the treatment of depression. The data suggest there is no stronger medicine than psychotherapy for depression. If we as therapists can learn to tolerate the emotional suffering of depression patients and help to guide them through it with specific psychotherapeutic strategies, as many as 80% will respond within 8 to 12 weeks of treatment, without drugs.

We are not suggesting that recovering from depression is a contest between pills and psychotherapy. It is our opinion that pills are not the answer to emotional, psychological, or spiritual problems; but we also reject the idea that psychotherapy has a monopoly on overcoming depression. Besides, there are so many kinds of psychotherapy that it can be misleading to speak of "psychotherapy" as if it were a single kind of human service.

For those desiring formal approaches, in addition to the multitude of psychotherapies, there are a variety of

Twelve-Step programs, inspirational religions, and psychospiritual workshops and retreats. We have already hinted at the variety of life experiences, including time itself, that heal depression.

It is our personal conviction that each person, hopefully with the support of loved ones, must find a way to make life meaningful.

But increasingly life is becoming a contest between pills—exemplified by Prozac—and life itself. People are giving up on life in favor of pills. They are abandoning the struggle to embrace life for the ease of swallowing a pill. There is an enormous cost attached to this choice.

One cost is a physical one—the effect on the brain and mind. This book has amply documented the physical threats entailed in taking drugs that disrupt the normal functions of the brain. We believe that there is a high likelihood of permanent brain dysfunction, especially when the drugs are taken for long periods of time.

But then there is a moral or psychological cost for the individual—the cost of giving up on oneself as a being with the capacity to triumph in life. In addition, there is the cost of blunting or otherwise impairing one's mental acuity at the very moment that one most needs it, at the personal crossroads during which despair vies with the opportunity for a great leap forward.

I'm often asked, "But what about taking a drug to get a jump start—to get enough energy to carry on?"

First, there is the scientific question: Do people really get jump starts from drugs? Some people do feel as if they get energized in a positive manner by taking an SSRI drug, and many psychiatrists claim that this frequently happens. The effect is probably no different from amphetamine or cocaine stimulation; the individual gets an abnormal burst of energy that may or may not turn out to be an advantage.

While some people might desire an artificial jolt, most people will experience it as a negative effect. Worse, taking one of the stimulant SSRIs may be risky. As we've seen, activating the depressed patient can *cause* suicide. Drugs that energize also have abuse potential and withdrawal problems. On balance, there is far more evidence for their capacity to cause mental aberrations than to ameliorate them.

Then there is the psychological challenge. We almost invariably become depressed when the old ways have stopped working—when we've come to a dead end in life. Sometimes the dead end seems caused by overwhelming tragedy, such as the breakup of a marriage or the death of a loved one. But almost always, if the despair becomes intense and unending, there's something else going on— problems restimulated from childhood, or attitudes or viewpoints that leave the person unprepared for life. At such a moment, revelations can occur, breathtaking changes can be made—life can evolve into something much better. This frequently happens in therapy, but thus far I've never seen it happen on a drug. And I've never seen it happen on a combination of drugs and therapy, because drug-taking, by its very nature, convinces the individual that he or she is at the mercy of forces beyond personal control. All psychoactive drugs disrupt brain and mental function, and hence self-awareness.

That point is worth stressing: The very taking of a pill becomes a sacrament of helplessness, a statement that the suffering is unendurable and beyond one's own means, that less suffering is preferable to an intact brain and a drug-free mind. Once drug-taking has begun, the individual is no longer likely to work his or her way out of the depression in a new and better way. At best, the drug-dulled or drug-driven individual adjusts or compulsively conforms.

THERE IS A POSITIVE SIDE OF DEPRESSION

Depression expresses energy. When a room is filled with oppressive black smoke, there's usually a fire nearby.

When patients tell me, in effect, that they are choking to death amid spiritual smoke, I tell them, metaphorically, "Where there's smoke, there's fire." The depth of their depression reflects the heat of passion burning within them. I explain, "The intensity of your suffering reflects the intensity of your life energy; imagine how fully you will live when you learn to use it creatively."

This is almost a mathematical equation: To the degree that a human being is capable of suffering deeply, to that same degree the human being is capable of a full, rich, exciting, and creative life. That's why people become "manic depressive"—their enormous frustrated energies drive them first into helpless gloom and then into equally futile euphoria. If a person has the energy—the vitality—to become "manic" or "depressive," then he or she also has the energy to live an extraordinarily rich and satisfying life. It's a matter of overcoming the dreadful legacy of childhood, especially self-hate and loathing, and learning to direct this remarkable energy into more productive channels.*

Sometimes people seem to think that, by discouraging the use of drugs, we demean the depth of their suffering. Nothing could be further from the truth. We ourselves have suffered deeply and known despair, and, in truth, all the people we love most dearly and know the best have gone through the same or similar experiences—our children, our parents, our friends, our clients and patients, our colleagues devoted to psychiatric reform and human freedom. Often the suffering has manifested itself as so-called clinical depression and at other times it has taken other forms. But for all the people we know and care about, the suffering, at one time or another, has seemed unendurable. Out of that suffering has come their unique understanding of life, their determination to care about

---

*For a critique of genetic and biological models for "manic depressive disorder," see Breggin 1991A.

themselves and others, and their will to live a spiritually rewarding life.

It's a truth communicated by Judeo-Christian and Eastern religions that the road to salvation must pass through suffering. The Buddhists say you cannot get to peace without passing through passion—passionate suffering. Have you ever read a biography or an autobiography of anyone whose life seemed worth recording—without discovering the depths of their emotional suffering? Offhand, we cannot recall anyone who has reached a moral or spiritual plateau of any consequence who hasn't done it at the cost of excruciating emotional pain. To rid ourselves of the option of suffering is to rid ourselves of ourselves.

DRUGS ARE THE TRULY DEMEANING APPROACH TO THERAPY

Phrases like "clinical depression" and "major depression" are truly demeaning expressions. They take profoundly important and often inevitable aspects of human existence, and reduce them to physical diseases. This approach robs us of the dignity to live a fully examined life and encourages us to solve life's most profound problems by putting ourselves in the hands of biological psychiatrists and their quick-fix technologies.

In response to what I'm saying, mental health professionals often say, "But there are extremes. Clinical depression is an extreme end of the continuum." Frankly, I'm not so sure about that. I see so much suffering around me that I don't know how to say one degree or another is somehow outside the bounds of normal.

But more important, who says that being extreme is being abnormal? That's how mental health professionals tend to think, but in their own lives they often prove that banality is another kind of failure. All of our personal heroes have been extremists—deeply passionate people who went through spiritual agony before finding their way and imprinting their values on the world. In fact, most of our personal friends are like that, too, even those who haven't yet found their way. Yet each and every one of them could have had their spiritual quest aborted by a psychiatric intervention. Instead of finding a new and higher road, they could have been left at the wayside as "psychiatric patients."

DRUGS, DEPRESSION, AND EMPATHY

Probably no other emotion is more highly developed or crucial in the human species than empathy. Empathy—a loving caring and concern for others—creates friendship, family, and society. It lies at the heart of all truly cooperative efforts. When especially heightened in an individual, it motivates the most creative and heroic actions. It is probably the single most important human quality.

Yet as the ultimate expression of our finely tuned brain and mind, empathy is the most vulnerable capacity. Lobotomy and newer forms of psychosurgery, for example, virtually eliminate it. Indeed, the production of relative degrees of indifference toward oneself and others is a central feature of the physical treatments in psychiatry. Prozac disrupts two of the neurotransmitters most involved in frontal-lobe function—serotonin and dopamine—and in that process can rob us of our sensitivity, self-awareness, and capacity to care or to love.

Put simply, the SSRIs are anti-empathic agents. That means they are anti-life—anti-human life in the fullest sense.

That Prozac and the other SSRIs blunt empathy may be the key to how they work at their best and at their worst. At their best, the person loses touch with himself or herself, becomes euphoric, and feels "better than ever." That's the ultimate Prozac cure. At their worst, the drug blunts empathy so that the person no longer has sympathy for himself or herself, or for anyone else. Then suicide and murder become possibilities.

In our violent society, some of the most shocking crimes are those committed by young people who appear to be totally without remorse or feeling for their victims. Many of us who work with children and adolescents find that our most important role is to help them rediscover empathy for themselves and others, and to help them reconnect to the world around them. Mind- and spirit-dulling drugs work against this.

It's empathy that makes us as human as we are, while helping us to manage our most violent feelings. We don't kill ourselves or others because we still see the human being in ourselves and others, and feel sympathy or caring. When our sense of connection is gone, then any kind of violence can be unleashed.

I have talked with people who have been tortured or been otherwise associated with torturers. They have told me their ultimate impression of people who torture other people. Torturers have lost touch with their own humanity. No longer able to care about themselves, they grow to hate others. Desperate to have any kind of feeling, they torture feelings out of others.

Rage reactions while under the influence of drugs have usually been explained as "disinhibition"—a loss of the customary controls imposed by the higher brain and with it a weakening of conscience. Biopsychiatrists and behaviorists have such a narrow vision of human nature, they imagine that it's inhibition that keeps us from harming each other. When we injure each other, they call it disinhibition. But it's not "inhibition" as much as human caring and empathy that keeps us from injuring each other.

Psychiatric drugs, by removing our fine-tuning toward ourselves and others, open the way to more destructive alternatives. In reducing emotional fine tuning, empathy is the first to go. This is because empathy is the most subtle, complex, and even delicate expression of our per-

Ɑnal fabric. To wash out our emotional static—those painful, discordant feelings—we must wash out ourselves as well.

One of the most commonly reported side effects on Prozac is a diminished sexuality, and often it does not seem to bother the afflicted person. The underlying defect may be the loss of interest in oneself and others. The Prozac user's alienation is frequently lamented by the friends, family, and loved ones of patients on Prozac—but not necessarily by the drug user.

Drugs are euthanasia of the soul, but a euthanasia applied at a heightened, if anguished, moment of life.

THE CONCEPT OF OVER-SENSITIVITY

Prozac is, as Peter Kramer claims, an anti-sensitivity drug. He devotes several cases and thousands of words to the subject of "over-sensitivity."

Nothing is more appalling than this concept of over-sensitivity. My patients frequently report to me on the first visit, "I'm too sensitive." It turns out that's what they were told by their parents, when their parents were abusing them: "You're too sensitive!" Nearly homicidal parents brutalize their children, watch them suffer, and then declare, "You're too sensitive." Teachers humiliate their students into tears and repeat the same theme. Abusive spouses justify their perpetrations by blaming the sensitivity of their victims.

There is no such thing as being too sensitive. There is such a thing as being insensitive, but it's not possible to be too aware, too responsive, too in touch. It is possible to be too injured and too humiliated, so that you wish you couldn't feel it anymore. In such cases, individuals need to understand and to overcome their vulnerability, to learn to defend themselves without sacrificing their emotional responsiveness, and to surround themselves with intimates who respect their feelings.

EMPATHY FOR THE CHILD YOU ONCE WERE

There's perhaps too much talk nowadays about the "inner child," but there's truth in the necessity of learning to care about the child that we once were, the real-life, breathing child who at age four or eight or twelve was suffering so much that the very idea of feeling anything became intolerable. Often in therapy, I encourage my patients to feel empathy for themselves as little children—not the metaphorical inner child, but the actual child, the one who was being beaten, molested, ridiculed, or abandoned, the one who wanted love and could not get it, the one who wanted safety and could find it nowhere.

Depressed people don't feel any empathy for themselves. You may think they do if they seem to complain or moan a lot, but it quickly becomes apparent that they hate and blame themselves. That's the opposite of empathy.

When deeply depressed persons do recall childhood, they will seem to feel empathy, not for themselves as abused children, but for their parents. "My dad had it rough, that's why he beat me." "My mom never got attention from anyone, that's why she never gave any to me." It goes on and on like that in therapy, as the depressed person feels—or seems to feel—for everyone but himself or herself.

Actually, the depressed person is feeling fear and guilt. It's not possible, from the child's viewpoint, to feel a genuinely deep caring for an abusive parent. What's being felt is terror—fear of abandonment and death. As Alice Miller has reminded us, the depressed child focuses on the parent in the vain hope of pleasing them enough to gain a little attention or to avoid dreadful punishment.

When a depressed adult at last feels empathy for himself or herself as a child, the depression begins to lift. Sorrow prevails as genuine feelings of pain and loss, but without the helplessness, and without the self-hate. Understanding replaces depression. When the adult has grasped his or her own plight as a child, self-hate becomes impossible. How can you hate yourself when you see what drove you into depression? How can you hate a five-year-old once you've gotten to know the child?

I want to emphasize I'm not talking about some mythical or metaphorical inner child; I'm talking about getting to know the real child who endured so much misery so many years ago. Once that loving connection is established between the adult and the child he or she once was, depression dissolves. Eventually, it may even be possible to empathize with the abusive parents, because they too were once abused children. But for this to be at all genuine, the adult must first empathize with himself or herself as a victimized youngster.

When people try to convince me that the depth of their suffering proves that they have a disease, I say just the opposite—that it proves they are alive, that there's still hope, and that their hope should be proportional to their pain. They are endowed with an extraordinary capacity for psychological and spiritual triumph. I do not say this glibly or in order to dismiss the pain or the enormously hard work of recovering and going on to live an even better life than previously seemed imaginable. Nor do I want to diminish the risks involved, including suicide. Life itself is a risk. But instead of trying to remove the risk with drugs—something that really cannot be done, anyway—I want to help people take on the challenge.

Peter Kramer's book, meanwhile, has done an enormous disservice by shifting the focus to "cosmetic psychopharmacology"—presumably a technological shortcut for people who want to find their real personalities the fast-food way. Taking stimulant drugs—from amphetamine and cocaine to the SSRIs—is not a good prescription for finding oneself. It would be considered a sad diversion from living a fully responsible and responsive life in a society that had sounder values. It would be held up to scorn and dismissed if we weren't running out of better values. But when we're already drugging more than a million children to avoid taking responsibility for *their* lives, why not drug ourselves to avoid taking responsibility for ourselves as well? The idea of cosmetic psychopharmacology can seem so appealing only in a world dominated by cosmetic values.

The concept of cosmetic psychopharmacology is doubly misleading and even destructive. People who turn to drugs in such a vain hope are themselves far more despairing than they are likely to admit. The despair may express itself as boredom or a kind of cynical or sophisticated alienation, but in reality, it goes deeper. That so many people feel the need for an artificial infusion of hope suggests that our society is failing to inspire us, and that we live lives of quiet desperation devoid of nurturing, comfort, and a sense of connection with others and with the world.

Finally, cosmetic psychopharmacology is misleading in a fashion that may truly come back to haunt us. Cosmetic implies superficial, as in smoothing out wrinkles with a tuck behind the ears. But there's nothing superficial about disrupting neurotransmission in the brain for days, weeks, months, or years on end. We are talking less about a cosmetic effect and more about a psychosurgical effect—a tampering with the very substance of the brain in a way that causes basic functions to go out of whack, in a way that drives neuronal receptors out of existence. It is euphemistic to talk of that as "cosmetic." The intent may be morally superficial, but the effect is physically, as well as morally, profound. Those who suffer drug-induced brain dysfunction can be rendered relatively unable to explore their human potential.

There aren't easy answers here. This isn't a quick-fix book. Rather, it's a book about the quick fix. We have no uncomplicated formulae to offer to the reader. Psychotherapy may help some people, but then it might not. Some psychotherapists are marvelously inspiring; many are certainly not. Some people dive enthusiastically into therapy like children throwing themselves into ocean breakers; others tiptoe up to their ankles as if entering shark-infested waters. The answer for each individual will vary. Our point is this: If you turn to drugs, you turn away from life. If you turn away from life, you sacrifice yourself even as you seek relief and healing.

As individuals we need moral support and inspiration. As a society, we need the same things. The goal in life, for us at least, is not mere pain reduction. Nor is it necessarily happiness. Many factors beyond our personal control affect our happiness. But we do believe in doing everything possible to fulfill our capacity to live, to love, to create, to contribute, to take responsibility and to grow; and then to encourage those around us to do the same. But we cannot, as individuals or a society, live by meaningful values unless we reject biological psychiatry, its fake medical diagnoses, and its drugs.

Expanding Our Vision of What It Means to Be a Person

More and more adults are deciding they are mentally ill and in need of Prozac. We don't want to endure discomfort within ourselves, let alone in others. Our concept of "normal behavior" grows more and more compressed. Conformity is being demanded at an earlier and earlier age. There are rapidly diminishing opportunities for self-expression and for experimenting with limits—for exercising individuality and testing oneself with others.

As we document in *The War Against Children*, there is a growing movement within psychiatry to do more medicating of children in the preschool years, and Prozac is joining Ritalin as the "drug of choice." At the same time, psychiatrists are more often saying that adult patients should remain on drugs for many years and often for a lifetime. Increasingly the elderly are being treated for depression with drugs and shock treatment, despite their obvious needs for a place of greater meaning in our society.[3] Psychiatry, not society, is becoming our guardian from the cradle to the grave.

The dangers of biopsychiatry for the individual and society cannot be exaggerated. Beyond causing physical side effects, drugs almost always blunt and confuse our emotional responses—our internal signal system. For the child or young adult, this means delaying and ultimately stunting the process of psychosocial growth and development during the years when self and identity are being formed. Our mettle is forged in the heat of human emotion and conflict, and drugs dampen and put out the fire.

For society, this expanding use of psychiatric diagnoses and drugs means that many of our most creative young people will never approach the fulfillment of their creative potential. Instead of struggling through the painful process of working out their personal relationship with themselves and others, they will—like the proverbial square pegs—be forced into round holes. Their edges will be shaved smooth in the process, and with it their uniqueness will be sacrificed.

For any age person, taking psychiatric drugs causes a more emotionally shallow life. It has been said that the unexamined life is not worth living. But what about the *unfelt* life? Is it a life at all?

LIVING BY MORE VITAL VALUES

The most common and crucial sources of disabling depression lie in childhood loses and abuses, but the intensity and persistence of depression is influenced by experiences in the larger society. What sort of social and educational resources does the community make available to emotionally injured children and their embattled families? What kind of guidance and inspiration can be found in community values? Does the future offer encouragement and hope to growing youngsters?

Environmentally oriented mental health professionals tend to focus on the individual and the "dysfunctional family" as the source of depression and other manifestations of despair. While this is an important approach, a more complete understanding takes into account the broader social context. When so many children are diagnosed with mental disorders including depression, we must ask about society's attitudes and policies toward its children. America, we believe, is grossly neglectful of its children. When so many women are diagnosed and treated for depression, we must ask similar questions about society's attitude toward them. For many women, the so-called real world is a hazardous and disappointing place.

We require more meaningful ways to live amid so much conflict and injustice, and, especially, we need to find personal values to sustain us in confronting and transforming an often bleak and dismaying reality.

While depression is in many ways an individual vulnerability and a private, personal affliction, it can be reinforced by our awareness and feeling of helplessness over the rampant injustices and tragedies in our world. Along with their perception of an unjust society, the overall alienation and lack of values felt by so many youngsters increases their vulnerability to depression.

Young people are especially likely to empathize with the suffering of others. They easily become discouraged about growing up in a world where children are malnourished amid excess food, where homeless people lie in gutters and atop grates in the richest country in the world, where whole ecosystems are destroyed on a daily basis, where massive pollution threatens us with everything from cancer to acid rain and global warming, where there is epidemic killing of other species—from songbirds to wolves and mountain gorillas. The most sensitive and empathic feel the greatest pain about the conditions around them.

Biological psychiatry—with its genetic and biological theories, drugs, and electroshock—is itself a depressing philosophy. It is no wonder that so many patients go from one drug to another, only to end up hospitalized for yet more toxic doses of drugs and electroshock. There is nothing inspiring about being psychiatrically diagnosed and subjected to physical treatment, and depressed people need, above all else, the inspiration to start living once again, this time in new and better ways.[4]

To lift oneself out of depression often requires learning new values that bring vitality and meaning to life: Facing the childhood hurts and adult disappointments that have made us vulnerable to depression; opening ourselves to suffering as a universal human experience, and moving through the painful emotions to a place of greater wisdom and acceptance; finding the courage to live in ways that we find truly satisfying and to pursue our most personal and idealistic goals; embracing the interconnectedness of ourselves and others, including all life forms and the earth, and deciding to reach out to life in more extraordinary ways; evolving ourselves mindfully toward making a greater contribution to the lives of those around us; and with eyes undimmed by the often tragic realities of existence, learning to love ourselves, others, and life itself.

Depression and love for life are incompatible, and love for life will always triumph when the individual finds the strength and courage to embrace it as the guiding principle of life.

Appendix

Books by the Breggins that provide further information on psychiatric drugs and disorders, and better alternatives:

Peter Breggin, M.D. *Toxic Psychiatry: Why Therapy, Empathy and Love Must Replace the Drugs, Electroshock and Biochemical Theories of the "New Psychiatry."* New York: St. Martin's Press, 1991.

Information and analyses regarding almost all psychiatric drugs and disorders not covered in *Talking Back to Prozac,* plus additional information on depression and how to treat it.

Peter R. Breggin, M.D. *Beyond Conflict: From Self-Help and Psychotherapy to Peacemaking.* New York, St. Martin's Press, 1993.

A comprehensive approach to resolving individual psychological difficulties, marital discord, and broader social conflict with special emphasis on the role of liberty and love.

Peter Breggin, M.D.; and **Ginger Ross Breggin**. *The War Against Children: How the Drugs, Programs, and Theories of the Psychiatric Establishment Are Threatening America's Children with a Medical "Cure" for Violence.* New York: St. Martin's Press, 1994.

The threat of biomedical (psychiatric) control of children and minorities, with extensive new information on childhood disorders and Ritalin.

To Learn About or to Join the Psychiatric Reform Movement

Children First!, Center for the Study of Psychiatry, 4628 Chestnut Street, Bethesda, MD 20814.

Children First! is the only national program that focuses on the dangers of biopsychiatric interventions into the lives of children and youth while supporting more caring alternatives. It needs your support to enlarge its national educational campaign against the wholesale diagnosing and drugging of America's children.

Children First! is a newly developed activity of the Center for the Study of Psychiatry. The center itself was founded in 1971 and is a nonprofit, tax-exempt research and educational institute devoted to reform in mental health. The center's Board of Directors and Advisory Council include more than a hundred leading psychiatrists and other mental health professionals, attorneys, patient advocates, psychiatric survivors, and members of Congress.

Peter R. Breggin, M.D., is executive director and Ginger Ross Breggin is director of research and education. John George, Ed.D., and Michael Valentine, Ph.D., are co-directors of *Children First!* and can be reached through the center.

Members receive periodic reports and the satisfaction of supporting these reform efforts on behalf of America's young people. Membership is open to anyone and the annual membership fee is $25.

The Prozac Survivors Support Group, Inc., Guy McConnell, National Director, 3080 Peach Avenue, No. 104, Clovis, CA 93612. Telephone: (209) 291-8661.

This organization brings together hundreds of victims of the adverse effects of Prozac and related drugs such as Zoloft and Paxil. Concerned families and friends also become members. It provides information, self-help, a support network, and conferences.

NARPA (National Association for Rights Protection and Advocacy), 587 Marshall Avenue, St. Paul, MN 55102. Telephone. (612) 224-7761.

NARPA is open to all people interested in supporting advocacy of patient and inmate rights, including both adults and children. You do not have to be a mental health professional or an activist in order to join. NARPA publishes a newsletter, *The Rights Tenet,* and holds an annual convention on patient rights and psychiatric reform, with workshops by lawyers, advocates, survivors, and reform-minded mental health professionals. It's worth joining to get the newsletter and to be reminded of the yearly conference, which is the best in the field. The Center for the Study of Psychiatry publishes a report in each NARPA newsletter and many Center Board and Advisory Council members usually give presentations at each annual conference. The annual NARPA membership fee is $20.

The National Association of Psychiatric Survivors (NAPS), P.O. Box 618, Sioux Falls, SD 57101.

If you have been damaged by psychiatry and want to join other survivors for moral support, political action, and the development of client-run alternatives, this organization is for you. Even if you are not a former patient, your membership and support is welcome. NAPS publishes a newsletter and can provide the addresses of local survivor groups around the United States and in many other countries. The annual membership fee is $25.

National Empowerment Center (NEC), 20 Ballard Road, Lawrence, MA 01843-1018. Telephone: 800-POWER-2-U. Fax: (508) 681-6426.

NEC is a new resource and information center for individuals and organizations concerned with empowering psychiatric survivors. It believes that all persons can take over and improve their lives. You can contact NEC to learn about the survivor movement and to locate resources in your community.

Dendron, PO Box 11284, Eugene, OR 97440. Telephone: (503) 341-0100.

Founded, edited, and published by David Oaks, this psychiatric survivor newsletter offers articles on psychiatric ppression, human rights, and self-help alternatives. It is highly recommended for staying in touch with what's happening in psychiatric reform and the survivor movement. The subscription rate is $12 for four issues.

To Obtain Legal Aid Against Psychiatric Abuse

The National Association of Protection and Advocacy Systems (NAPAS), 900 Second Street, NE, Suite 211, Washington, DC 20002. Telephone: (202) 408-9514.

If you are or have recently been an inmate subjected to abusive psychiatric treatment in any institution, public or private, and need help in protecting your rights, you can contact NAPAS. It can provide you with the address and phone number of federally funded Protection and Advocacy agencies in your state. Many of these state agencies are doing good work supporting patient rights and investigating violations. The services are free. They may be able to provide referrals to sympathetic private attorneys as well.

To Find a Psychotherapist

The American Academy of Psychotherapists (AAP), PO Box 607, Decatur, GA 30031. Telephone: (404) 299-6336.

The AAP central office can provide names from among its several hundred members, some of whom may live in your area, including psychologists, psychiatrists, social workers, counselors, and other professionals. AAP members are trained and experienced in psychotherapy and have themselves undergone psychotherapy. Get several names and shop carefully for a person with whom you feel comfortable and confident. Membership in any organization does not guarantee that an individual is ethical or competent. AAP is not affiliated with the Center for the Study of Psychiatry or any other psychiatric reform organization, and membership in AAP indicates nothing about a psychotherapist's views on drugs or other issues. It is up to the individual seeking help to question any potential therapist about his or her approach and values.

To Find a Full-Service Clinic

San Joaquin Psychotherapy Center, 3114 Willow Avenue, Clovis, CA 93612. Telephone: (209) 292-7572.

Kevin McCready, Ph.D., is founder and director of the center, which provides a broad spectrum of daytime and evening services that includes psychotherapy as well as group, recreational, music and art therapy. The orientation is psychosocial; psychiatric drugs are not encouraged, and patients will be helped to withdraw from drugs if they wish. There are no overnight or hospital services, but individuals may find their own accommodations while working with the clinic during daytime and evening hours.

Commonly Used Sources of Drug Information in Psychiatry

The following books can provide some useful information, but they suffer from biases toward biopsychiatry.

American Psychiatric Association. *Treatments of Psychiatric Disorders* (four volumes). Washington, D.C.: American Psychiatric Association, 1989.

American Psychiatric Association Task Force Report. *Benzodiazepine Dependency, Toxicity and Abuse.* Washington, D.C.: American Psychiatric Association, 1990.

Goodman, Alfred, Louis Goodman, Theodore Rall, Murad Ferid. *The Pharmacological Basis of Therapeutics.* New York: Macmillan, 1991.

Gorman, Jack. *The Essential Guide to Psychiatric Drugs.* New York: St. Martin's Press, 1990.

Kaplan, Harold, and Benjamin Sadock, eds. *Comprehensive Textbook of Psychiatry.* Baltimore, MD: Williams & Wilkins, 1989.

Physicians' Desk Reference (PDR). Oradell, NJ: Medical Economics, 1994. Published annually.

Talbott, John, Robert Hales, and Stuart Yudofsky, eds. *Text-*

book of Psychiatry. Washington, D.C.: American Psychiatric Press, 1988.

USP DI. *Drug Information for the Health Care Professional.* Rockville, MD: U.S. Pharmacopeial Convention, 1994. Published annually.

How to File an Adverse Drug Reaction Report with the FDA

If you or someone you know has suffered a serious adverse or negative reaction to a medication or medical device, the FDA's new MEDWATCH report can be filled out and sent to the agency. It is probably most convincing and effective for physicians to file MEDWATCH reports, but anyone can do so.

To apply for the MEDWATCH report form, contact:

MEDWATCH
The FDA Medical Products Reporting Program
Food and Drug Administration
5600 Fishers Lane
Rockville, MD 20852-9787
Or Fax to: 1-800-FDA-0178.

Notes

1. Should We Listen to Prozac?

1. Rimer, December 13, 1993.
2. Tobias, 1990.
3. Figures from Freudenheim, 1990. Lilly's top seller at the time was Ceclor, followed by Prozac, Humulin Insulin, and Keflex and Keftabs. Lilly also makes Darvon.
4. These figures are taken from a March 26, 1990, *Newsweek* article by Geoffrey Cowley and presumably were obtained from Eli Lilly. No government agency or other independent body collects this data.
5. For a critique of Kramer, see Rothman, 1994.
6. Cowley, February 7, 1994.
7. Cowley, February 7, 1994.
8. The term essentially means "imagined ugliness."
9. Eagan, 1994, cites 600 patients. Brandt, 1994, cites 700. Goodwin has told me that the figure is now up to 800. The *Oprah* show was actually filmed on February 15, 1994.
10. See Miller, M., March 31, 1994.
11. Eli Lilly and Company, 1992
12. Breggin, 1992h.
13. See Breggin, 1991a, for a review of the minor tranquilizers such as Valium, Librium, Xanax, Ativan, and Klonopin. For an earlier critical analysis, see Bargmann *et al.*, 1983.

A Primer on How Prozac Is Supposed to Work

1. For a summary of Prozac's effect from the viewpoint of a Lilly researcher, see Fuller, 1986.
2. Wamsley *et al.*, 1987. Prozac brought about a compensatory decrease in the number of adrenergic receptors in the brain. This indicates it was stimulating the system.
3. For neuroanatomical details of the serotonin system, see Tork and Hornung, 1990.
4. For example, see Patraglia *et al.*, 1986, and Stark *et al.*, 1985.
5. Gilman *et al.*, 1991, p. 593.
6. *Psychiatric News,* February 4, 1994.
7. Most of these older antidepressants are discussed in *Toxic Psychiatry* (Breggin, 1991a), as well as in any textbook of psychiatry. The following tricyclics block the reuptake of both norepinephrine and serotonin, and therefore can at times produce serotonergic effects similar to the SSRIs: amitriptyline (Elavil, Endep), desipramine (Norpramin, Pertofrane), doxepin (Sinequan, Adapin), imipramine (Tofranil, Janimine, SK-Pramine), nortriptyline (Pamelor, Aventyl), protriptyline (Vivactil), and clomipramine (Anafranil). The neuroleptic-antidepressant amoxapine (Asendin) also blocks the uptake of both norepinephrine and serotonin. The four most potent blockers of serotonin reuptake among these drugs are clomipramine, followed by amitriptyline and imipramine, and then amoxapine. Trazodone (Desyrel), which is chemically unique, blocks the reuptake of serotonin, with little impact on norepinephrine. The tetracyclic maprotiline (Ludiomil) blocks norepinephrine but not serotonin. The tricyclic trimipramine (Surmontil) and the monocyclic buproprion (Wellbutrin) do not block the uptake of either neurotransmitter. The monoamine oxidase inhibitors (MAOIs), isocarboxazid (Marplan), phenelzine (Nardil), selegiline (Eldepryl, not approved for depression) and tranylcypromine (Parnate), are not reuptake blockers, but can cause serotonergic stimulation, producing stimulant adverse effects similar to Prozac and other SSRIs. The serotonergic stim-

ulation can be very dangerous when MAOIs are mistakenly combined with other drugs that stimulate the same system, such as tryptophan and tricyclic antidepressants. From this list, it becomes apparent what a wide variety of drugs become labeled antidepressants, leading to an equally wide variety of speculations about how or why they work.

8. Quoted in Sherman, February 1994, p. 3.
9. In my books *Psychiatric Drugs* (1983) and *Toxic Psychiatry* (1991), as well as in articles and book chapters, I have tried to show that all psychiatric drugs disable the brain and that none improves its function.

3. The Real Story Behind Prozac's Approval by the FDA

1. For a good discussion of placebo, see Greenberg and Fisher, 1989.
2. Food and Drug Administration, March 28, 1985, pp. 3–4, and elsewhere.
3. In a critical examination of placebo washout, Fred Reimherr from the University of Utah and his colleagues found that in some cases, at least, the methodology would "artificially suppress the level of placebo-induced improvement," a result that would artificially improve the performance of the drug by comparison. Overall, Reimherr found that the use of placebo washout had "unpredictable, possibly confounding" effects.
4. For advocates of Prozac for children and adolescents, see Baker, 1993; Fieve, 1994.
5. Food and Drug Administration, October 3, 1988, p. 27.
6. *Ibid.* The summary begins on page 18 of the document.
7. *Ibid.,* March 28, 1985, p. 68, for comment on comparison to imipramine studies.
8. Cited in Office of the Inspector General, 1992.
9. See Kline *et al.,* 1993.
10. The improvement was on a scale called "Patient's Global Depressions."
11. Food and Drug Administration, December 30, 1985, p. 13.
12. Fieve, 1994, pp. ix–x.

13. If 33.3 percent (one-third) of Fieve's Prozac patients drop out, that leaves 66.7 percent. If there is improvement in 70 percent of the remaining 66.7 percent, that's an improvement rate of 46.6 percent, which is not usually significant when compared to placebo.

14. Greenberg *et al.,* 1992; Greenberg and Fisher, 1989; and Fisher and Greenberg, 1993. This Seymour Fisher is a different person from the Seymour Fisher who coauthored Fisher, Bryant, and Kent, 1993.

4. The Real Story Behind Prozac's Side Effects

1. Thompson, 1994.

2. Kapit, December 7, 1986.

3. Kapit, March 4, 1988.

4. The symptoms we have listed occurred more frequently than those associated with placebo. The difference between the frequency associated with the drug and that associated with the placebo is sometimes thought to reflect the actual frequency associated with the drug itself. Thus, when 20 percent of patients get "headache" from the drug and 15 percent get it from the placebo, it is assumed that 5 percent is the rate of "headache" produced by the actual drug effect. But the side effects reported with drugs are likely to be more intense or threatening than those associated with placebo. That is, the drug-induced headaches may have been far more severe than those produced by the placebo.

5. Boyer and Feighner, 1992.

6. Humphries *et al.,* 1990.

7. Brandes *et al.,* 1992.

8. Ahtee and Eriksson, 1972.

9. Myers and Veale, 1968.

10. Sternbach, 1991, presents cases and reviews the extensive literature.

11. To make matters worse, the authors point out, the doses of antidepressants were small and they were administered only once a day, and therefore could "underestimate the full impact of this interaction" when both medications are given under routine treatment conditions.

We are grateful to Guy McConnell, national director of the Prozac Survivors Support Group, for drawing our attention to this important paper.

12. Tricyclics begin to have increased adverse effects when they rise only a little above their recommended maximum levels, and become very toxic when their levels are doubled or quadrupled. The commonly used tricyclic, amitriptyline or Elavil, for example, can be toxic when the normal high for its blood level is merely doubled from 250 ng/ml to 500 ng/ml. The other tricyclics become extremely toxic when their maximum therapeutic levels are increased a mere fourfold from 250 ng/ml to 1000 ng/ml. Another tricyclic, nortriptyline or Aventyl/Pamelor, has a small "therapeutic window." That is, its therapeutic effect is reduced once it reaches a level slightly above its recommended one. The data summarized here can be found in most handbooks of drug treatment, *e.g.*, Maxmen, 1991.

13. Baron *et al.,* 1988. Down-regulation of adrenergic receptors was greatly increased in rapidity and intensity by the combination.

14. For a more complete discussion of tardive dyskinesia and related disorders, see American Psychiatric Association, 1980 and 1992; Breggin, 1991a.

15. Breggin, 1983a, 1990a, 1991a, 1993c.

16. *The Medical Letter,* September 7, 1990.

17. See Reccoppa *et al.,* 1990, and Meltzer *et al.,* 1979.

18. Weiner and Luby, 1983, published an early report of tardive akathisia. Gualtieri and Sovner, 1989, reviewed the subject in depth, cited studies with prevalence rates of 13 to 18 percent, and called it "a significant public health issue." Nonetheless, the drug companies and the FDA have ignored it.

19. Also see Schmidt, 1987.

20. Ricaurte *et al.,* 1983.

21. Wong and Bymaster, 1981; Wong *et al.,* 1985; Wamsley *et al.,* 1987. At lower doses, there were both increases and decreases in receptor density in various areas of the brain, according to Wamsley, indicating the complexity. Also, see Fuller *et al.,* 1974. Down-regulation as an adaptation to overstimulation seems to occur in most or all known receptor systems.

22. The neuroleptics suppress dopamine neurotransmission.

The deprived dopamine receptors become hyperactive and proliferate in number. This process can become permanent and probably plays a prominent role in the production of tardive dyskinesia. See Breggin, 1983a and 1991a, or any textbook of psychiatry, such as Talbott *et al.*, 1988.

23. A sample includes Settle and Settle, 1984; Chouinard and Steiner, 1986; Turner *et al.*, 1985; Lebegue, 1987. For a case induced by Zoloft, see Laporta *et al.*, 1987.

24. Impairment was found by Murray *et al.*, 1993, and none was found by Fudge *et al.*, 1990.

25. I have developed and documented the brain-disabling principle in my professional articles (Breggin, 1980, 1981a&b, 1983b) and in two medical textbooks (Breggin, 1979 and 1983a), as well as in a more readily available source, *Toxic Psychiatry,* 1991.

26. Documented in detail in Breggin, 1983, and Breggin, 1991a. The continuum of indifference and apathy to a more severe rousable stupor is evaluated more thoroughly as the "deactivation" continuum in Breggin, 1993c.

27. Lee, 1993.

28. See, for example, Baghurst, 1992, and Thompson, 1992.

29. For example, Abrams, 1988, pp. 159–61.

30. The possible psychosurgical delivery of serotonin is described in a book by Rodgers, 1992, p. 106.

5. Drug Addiction and Abuse

1. For a comparison, see Gilman et al., pp. 508 and 510.

2. The history of Darvon up to this point in time is taken from Hughes and Brewin, 1979.

3. Good historical discussions of cocaine and amphetamines can be found in Consumers Union Report, 1972. For more detail in regard to cocaine, see Grinspoon and Bakalar, 1976.

4. See Consumers Union Report, 1972, for a summary, and Jones, 1953, Chapter 6, "The Cocaine Episode," for the details.

5. Reviewed in Grinspoon and Hedblom, 1975, Chapter 8.

6. It was published two years later.

7. Summarized in Cole, 1972. Original data in Balter and Levine, 1969.
8. The quote is from Grinspoon and Bakalar, 1985.
9. Breggin, 1992e.
10. World Health Organization, 1957. Cited in Grinspoon and Hedblom, 1975, p. 157.
11. A variety of animal studies show that the more seroto-nergic activity, the lower the need for amphetamines, and vice versa. See Lyness, 1983; Leccese and Lyness, 1984, and Lyness *et al.,* 1980.
12. Louie *et al.,* 1994.
13. Kramer, 1993, p. 265.
14. Kramer, 1993, p. 231.
15. Kramer, 1993, p. 359.
16. Gilman *et al.,* 1991, p. 1646.

6. *Drug-Induced Paranoia, Violence, Depression, and Suicide*

1. Breggin, 1992h.
2. Smith, 1972.
3. Scher, 1967.
4. Grinspoon and Hedblom, 1975, discuss these psychological effects.
5. Randrup and Munkvad, 1972.
6. Spotts and Spotts, 1980, p. 369.
7. Spotts and Spotts, 1980, p. 372.
8. Spotts and Spotts, 1980, p. 370.
9. Also see Ellinwood, 1971.
10. Ellinwood, 1971.
11. In the *DSM-III-R* (American Psychiatric Association, 1987), amphetamine *intoxication* is characterized by "Maladaptive behavioral changes, e.g., fighting, grandiosity, hypervigilance, psychomotor agitation, impaired judgment, impaired social or occupational functioning." In amphetamine *delirium,* according to the diagnostic manual, "Violent and aggressive behavior is common, and restraint may be required." Stimulant *delusional disorder* may "induce aggressive or violent action against 'enemies.' "
12. Gawin and Ellinwood, 1989, p. 1224.

13. Randrup and Munkvad, 1972, for an early review. For brief recent summaries, see Frances and Franklin, 1988, or Jaffe, 1989. For more detailed summaries, see Hoffman and Lefkowitz, 1991, and other relevant chapters in Gilman *et al.*, 1991, as well as Gawin and Ellinwood, 1989.

14. Some researchers believe a combination of serotonergic and dopaminergic effects, or serotonergic effects alone, may cause drug-induced psychosis (Hoffman and Lefkowitz, 1991, pp. 211–212), while others focus on serotonin alone.

15. We are grateful to Benjamin Breggin for drawing this interesting book to our attention.

7. Can Prozac Cause Violence and Suicide?

1. Food and Drug Administration, September 20, 1991A.
2. Blodgett, 1990.
3. Inquisition, 1989.
4. Marcus, February 7, 1991; Brataas, 1991.
5. *Los Angeles Times,* 1990.
6. Kifner, 1990.
7. McLaughlin, 1990.
8. *The Courier-Journal* (Louisville, KY), 1990.
9. Nathanson, 1990.
10. *Los Angeles Daily Journal,* 1990.
11. Marcus, February 7, 1991.
12. Brataas, 1991. The teacher pleaded guilty to burglary, and the other charges were dropped.
13. Charles, 1991.
14. Limbacher, 1991.
15. Rosenlind, July 23 and October 26, 1991. Also, Turner, 1991.
16. *Press-Courier* (Oxnard, CA), 1991.
17. Duggan, 1991.
18. Burns, 1991.
19. Timmins, 1991.
20. Associated Press, November 8, 1991. Also see Schwartz, 1991.
21. Eddy and Lipsher, 1991.
22. Tolliver, 1991.
23. *News & Record* (Halifax, VA), 1991.

24. Reinbrech, 1991; also see Wise, 1991.
25. Baird, 1991. She claimed she had fallen asleep at the wheel due to the drug, but she also behaved impulsively, fleeing from the scene.
26. Hilgers, 1991.
27. Pimsleur, 1991.
28. Hinmon and Scruggs, 1991.
29. Swadish, 1991.
30. *Daily Courier* (West Canada), 1991.
31. *Cincinnati Enquirer,* 1991.
32. Marcus, February 7, 1991.
33. Tolliver, 1991, and Marcus, 1991. The description of the woman's feelings were provided during an interview I had with Bonnie Leitsch, who attended her trial.
34. See Food and Drug Administration, September 20, 1991. Also Angier, 1991, and Associated Press, January 30, 1991.
35. Graedon and Graedon, 1991.
36. *Salt Lake Tribune,* 1991.
37. *Reporter & Messenger* (Rockdale, TX), 1991.
38. Belli, 1991.
39. Rosen, 1992.
40. Mooty, 1991.
41. Toups, 1991.
42. Toups, 1991.
43. Bunch and Trotter, 1991.
44. Vosburgh, 1991.
45. Brataas, 1991, and Cassano, 1991.
46. Cassada, 1991.
47. Duran, 1992. The January 1992 story describes a 1991 crime.
48. Saterfield, December 5, 1991.
49. Higham, 1991.
50. His daughter says that at no time had he voiced suicidal ideas. He was much too afraid of pain to have chosen self-inflicted knife wounds as a way to commit suicide.
51. Teicher makes the same point in his 1990 testimony, p. 83.
52. The German package insert developed by the BGA, the German counterpart of the FDA, states "there are reports of the following health problems which occurred during treatment with Fluctin [Prozac], although Fluctin may not have been the cause." Among them are "suicidal thoughts and aggressive behavior."

The most commonly used reference source by Canadian doctors is the *Compendium of Pharmaceuticals and Specialties (CPS)*, published by the Canadian Pharmaceutical Association. Its 1993 edition introduces its summary of adverse effects by saying that each of them was reported "on at least one occasion." It includes "hostility" and under "Rare," it adds the following: "antisocial reaction," "suicidal ideation," and "violent behaviors."

53. Only one was an inpatient. The total of all patients treated with Prozac was 172. Teicher, 1990.

54. Miller, 1990, pointed out that some of the doses were relatively high at 80 mgs. per day, and two had been continued on Prozac after a rash appeared. Some of the patients had their doses increased after developing symptoms of central nervous system side effects. And all but one patient had experienced suicidal ideation in the past. The several letters by Teicher's group defend against this criticism.

55. As cited in Kilgore, 1991, Rosenbaum—in apparent contradiction to the results of his study—said he was now including the possibility of rare behavioral effects in his discussions about side effects with patients.

56. The Harvard team presented their reanalysis of the data in 1990, but for the most detail see Teicher *et al.,* 1993.

57. The study cited by Teicher is Avery and Winokur, 1978.

58. Food and Drug Administration, September 20, 1991, p. 290.

59. Food and Drug Administration, September 20, 1991A, p. 126ff.

60. Teicher, November 15, 1990, p. 6.

61. Teicher *et al.,* December 1990, also made the point that their own original six patients seem to present with "a very clear organic flavor," meaning that they had drug-induced brain dysfunction, as in a toxic state.

62. Food and Drug Administration, September 20, 1991A, p. 281.

63. Public citizen, May 23, 1991; also Reuters, May 24, 1991.

64. Teicher *et al.,* November 1990. Also discussed in Teicher, November 15, 1990, p. 51.

65. Dasgupta, 1990; Masand *et al.,* 1991; Hoover, 1990—retracted by Hoover, 1991.

66. Masand *et al.,* 1991, followed by Dewan and Masand, 1991.

67. Papp and Gorman, 1990, hypothesized that the mental abnormality might be due to an initial surge in serotonergic neurotransmission, before desensitization of the receptors took place. Their comment underscores the lack of understanding about Prozac's impact on the brain even among sophisticated pharmacologically oriented psychiatrists. The initial impact of Prozac is to shut down the serotonergic system. See ahead in this chapter.

68. For example, Chouinard and Steiner, 1986; Jerome, 1991; Lensgraf and Favazza, 1990.

69. Hersh, 1991; Mandalos and Szarek, 1990. In neither case did the paranoia escalate to violence.

70. *Lancet,* Editorial, 1990.

71. Drake and Ehrlich, 1985; Fava and Rosenbaum, 1990, and Korn *et al.,* 1992; Kalda, 1993.

72. Food and Drug Administration, September 20, 1991A, p. 190ff.

73. Food and Drug Administration, September 20, 1991A, pp. 196–197.

74. Stimmel *et al.,* 1991.

75. Teicher *et al.,* 1993, also cite this frequently described phenomenon.

76. Keckich, 1978; Shear *et al.,* 1983; Drake and Ehrlich, 1985; and Crowner *et al.,* 1990.

77. Rothschild and Locke, 1991, observed these reactions in only three of 1500 patients. They attribute this relatively low incidence "to our lowering of fluoxetine dose when side effects develop and to the prompt recognition and treatment of akathisia." There is no better illustration of the need to inform physicians of the dangers of Prozac.

78. The Public Citizen Health Research Group lists barbiturates such as phenobarbital; minor tranquilizers such as diazepam (Valium) and triazolam (Halcion); heart drugs containing reserpine (Serpasil); beta-blockers such as propranolol (Inderal); blood pressure drugs such as clonidine (Catapres), methyldopa (Aldomet), and prazosin (Minipress); cardiac antiarrhythmic drugs such as disopyramide (Norpace); ulcer drugs such as cimetidine (Tagamet) and ranitidine (Zantac); antiparkinsonian drugs such as levodopa (Dopar) and bromocriptine (Parlodel); corticosteroids such as cortisone and prednisone; anticonvulsants such as phenytonin (Dilantin), ethosuximide (Zarontin)

and primidone (Mysoline); antibiotics such as cycloserine (Seromycin), isoniazid (INH), ethionamide (Trecator-SC), and metronidazole (Flagyl); diet pills such as amphetamines (during withdrawal); painkillers and arthritis drugs such as pentazocine (Talwin), indomethacin (Indocin), and ibuprofen (Motrin, Rufen, Advil, Nuprin); and various other drugs including metrizamide (Ampaque, used for diagnosing slipped discs) and disulfiram (Antabuse, used for alcoholism). Consistent with their support of the stronger psychiatric drugs, they do not list the neuroleptic drugs, such as Haldol, Thorazine, Mellaril, Prolixin, and Navane, which can cause depression. Nor do they list lithium and the tricyclic antidepressants, such as Tofranil and Elavil, all of which have been implicated in causing depression.

See *Journal of Clinical Psychiatry,* December 1993, for long-delayed professional recognition that neuroleptic drugs often turn patients into zombies. This was obvious from when they were first used and has frequently been reported by survivors of the treatment (see Breggin, 1983a, 1991a).

79. See Breggin, 1983a, 1990a, 1991a, and 1993c.

80. See Teicher *et al.,* 1993.

81. See, for example, Higley *et al.,* 1992 and 1993 (rhesus monkey studies at NIH); Kruesi *et al.,* 1990 and 1993 (impulsive child studies at NIMH); Brown, S., and van Praag, 1991, and Brown, G. and Linnoila, 1990 (the whole spectrum of possible serotonin-related disorders); Apter *et al.,* 1986, for suicide and violence. Touchette, 1994, cites the opinions of current researchers.

82. See Touchette, 1994.

83. Kotulak, 1993 (five articles in the *Chicago Tribune*).

84. See Fuller and Wong, 1977, as well as the other Fuller references, and Clemens *et al.,* 1977. Also see de Montigny *et al.,* 1990.

85. The percentages are from Wamsley *et al.,* 1987. Also see Wong and Bymaster, 1981, Wong *et al.,* 1985, and Wexler *et al.,* 1989.

86. Pennisi, 1994; Barinaga, 1994.

87. Welner, 1989.

88. See Wong *et al.,* 1974, and Stark *et al.,* 1985.

89. See, for example, Breggin, 1991a; Gualtieri, 1991; Mann and Kapur, 1991; and Wirshing *et al.,* 1992.

90. Fuller and Beasley, 1991, and Fuller, in a letter to me, January 7, 1992.

91. Blier *et al.,* 1988. In a telephone call, Blier disagreed with my interpretation of his research, which was funded in part by Eli Lilly. At issue is the reduction of firing activity of ascending nerve pathways presented in Table 1 (p. 250) and called "small but significant" (text p. 252).

92. Bymaster and Wong, August 20, 1974.

8. Pushing Drugs in America

1. Breggin, 1993a; Gilman *et al.,* 1991; United States General Accounting Office, 1990.

2. Gilman *et al.,* 1991, p. 78; also see Breggin, 1993a.

3. See United States General Accounting Office, 1990, and Breggin, 1993a, as well as Breggin, 1991a.

4. Smith, 1994.

5. Food and Drug Administration, September 20, 1991A, pp. 141 and 150. The FDA's data is compromised by the fact that prior to January 1989 suicide attempts were not part of their reporting dictionary of items, and got lumped instead under overdose or psychotic depression. See p. 141.

6. Breggin, 1992e.

7. Food and Drug Administration, September 20, 1991A, p. 147.

8. Described by Wohl, 1984.

9. See Breggin and Breggin, 1994.

10. See Arno and Feiden, 1992; Breggin, 1991a and 1993a; Carlson, 1992; *Journal of the American Medical Association,* 1992; Karel, 1993; Reuters, 1992; United States General Accounting Office (GAO), 1992; Valentine, 1990.

11. Carlson, 1992. AARP stands for the American Association of Retired Persons.

12. Reuters, November 23, 1992. Also see Kolata, 1992.

13. Hunt and Frankel, 1991; Karel, 1993; *Psychiatric Times,* 1991; Rosenthal, 1991.

14. Breggin, 1991a.

15. Breggin, 1992g and 1991a.

16. The letter from APA was written by its medical director, Melvin Sabshin, 1992, in response to my letter to the *New*

York Times. The letter from Upjohn was written by Jonas, 1992.

17. A recent scandal disclosed outright bribes of officials at the FDA by industries pushing generic drugs. See Valentine, 1990. Also see Breggin 1991A, p. 362.

18. *Journal of the American Medical Association,* 1992.

19. Food and Drug Administration, September 20, 1991B.

20. Food and Drug Administration, September 16, 1991.

21. Fishman, 1990.

22. For detailed documentation, see Breggin, 1991a.

23. Gubin, 1993.

24. Tanouye, 1993.

25. See Breggin, 1991a for documentation.

26. FAES provides a variety of services to NIH—courses, special awards, music and lecture series, artwork displays, and salary supplements (drug company–funded) to postdoctoral-level scientists "whose stipends are otherwise inadequate." The four courses FAES sponsored confirm its biomedical orientation: endocrinology, pathology, medical genetics, and psychopharmacology. The absence of psychosocial approaches is noteworthy. FAES also provides a "social and academic center" on 1.5 acres of prime land adjacent to NIH.

27. This is a recent discovery. We are looking into the total amounts awarded by drug companies to Rapoport and others.

28. Foundation for Advanced Education in the Sciences (FAES), 1993.

29. William Styron, 1993, describes how "a gentleman who identified himself as the acting director of the National Institute of Mental Health" edged him away from the microphone at a press conference following his presentation during "A Conference With William Styron." Styron had begun to criticize Prozac, and Eli Lilly was sponsoring the conference. See Karel, 1993.

30. Cockburn, 1994.

31. Kosterlitz, 1987.

32. Schwartz, 1993; Hilts, 1993.

33. Cockburn, 1992.

34. Associated Press, October 12, 1992.

35. See Specter, 1990 for the cause of the drug-related illness and Manders, 1992 for criticism of the ban.

36. Marcus, April 9, 1991.
37. Marcus, April 9, 1991; Marcus and Lambert, 1991; Reuters, June 5, 1991.
38. Reuters, June 5, 1991.
39. In *Toxic Psychiatry,* for example, I focus on Upjohn, the maker of Halcion and Xanax, rather than on Eli Lilly.

9. How and Why to Stop Taking Psychiatric Drugs

1. Electroshock has made a comeback and is currently given to up to 100,000 patients per year in the United States. I review the subject in *Toxic Psychiatry* (1991a) and present an updated criticism in *Readings* (1992f). For further criticism of shock, see Breggin, 1979 and 1981a. In addition to any textbook of psychiatry, for advocacy of shock see Abrams, 1988; but be aware that among his professorial credentials, Abrams fails to mention that he is president of a shock company and makes 50 percent of his income from it (documented in Breggin, 1991a).
2. Iatrogenic denial is described in detail in Breggin, 1983b, and also in Breggin, 1991a.
3. See Breggin, 1991a, and Breggin and Breggin, 1994, for discussions of the drugging of children.
4. See Breggin, 1991a.
5. Paradoxical effects of sedative tranquilizers are discussed in Breggin, 1991a.
6. Breggin, 1991a; Karel, 1991; Hunt and Frankel, 1991.

10. Understanding and Overcoming Depression

1. The NIMH estimates are drawn from an article by Regier *et al.,* 1988, that was published as part of a carefully constructed media campaign—the NIMH "Depression Awareness, Recognition, and Treatment Program" (also called D/ART). The NIMH brochure for the D/ART was widely distributed by Eli Lilly with the manufacturer's logo and name on it.
2. Reviewed in Breggin, 1991a and 1992a.

3. The causes and treatment of depression in the elderly is discussed in Breggin, 1991a.
4. Joanna Macy, Thich Nhat Hanh, Charlene Spretnak, John Seed, and Wendell Berry explore both the pain of people and the earth out of balance, and various paths that can be taken to bring greater harmony into one's personal life and the world at large. Macy, Hanh, and Spretnak have chapters in Eppsteiner, 1988; see Seed *et al.*, 1988, for Macy; see Berry, 1977. P. Breggin, 1992a, describes G. Breggin's overall concept of shared values, as well as his own application of the values of liberty and love to practical living.

Bibliography

Abrams, Richard (1988). *Electroconvulsive Therapy.* New York: Oxford University Press.

Achenbach, Joel (1992, May 6). "Mind Over Gray Matter? Psychiatrists Debate Power of the Pill." *Washington Post,* p. B1.

Ahtee, L., and K. Eriksson (1972). "5-Hydroxytryptamine and 5-Hydroxindolylacetic Acid Content in Brain of Rat Strains Selected for Their Alcohol Intake." *Physiology and Behavior,* 8:123–126.

American Medical Association (1966). "Report of the Committee on Alcoholism and Addiction and Council on Mental Health." *Journal of the American Medical Association,* 197: 193–197.

American Psychiatric Association (1980). *Tardive Dyskinesia: Report of the American Psychiatric Association Task Force on Late Neurological Effects of Antipsychotic Drugs.* Washington, D.C.: American Psychiatric Association.

American Psychiatric Association (1987). *Diagnostic and Statistical Manual of Mental Disorders (Third Edition, Revised) (DSM-III-R).* Washington, D.C.: American Psychiatric Association.

American Psychiatric Association (1989). *Treatments of Psychiatric Disorders.* Washington, D.C.: American Psychiatric Association.

American Psychiatric Association (1992). *Tardive Dyskinesia: A Task Force Report.* Washington, D.C.: American Psychiatric Association.

Angier, Natalie (1990, August 16). "Eli Lilly Facing Million-

Dollar Suits on Its Antidepressant Drug Prozac." *New York Times,* p. 399.

Angier, Natalie (1991, February 7). "Suicidal Behavior Tied Again to Drug." *New York Times,* p. B15.

Antonuccio, David (1993, August 23). "Psychotherapy vs. Medication for Depression: Challenging the Conventional Wisdom." Presented at the Annual Convention of the American Psychological Association, Toronto, Canada.

Apter, Alan, Serena-Lynn Brown, Martin L. Korn, and Herman M. van Praag (1986). "Serotonergic Parameters of Aggression and Suicide." In Mann, J. John, and Michael Stanley (eds.): *Psychobiology of Suicidal Behavior.* New York: New York Academy of Sciences, Chapter 12, pp. 284–301.

Armstrong, Louise (1993). *And They Call It Help: The Psychiatric Policing of America's Children.* New York: Addison-Wesley Publishing Co.

Arno, Peter S., and Karyn L. Feiden (1992). *Against the Odds: The Story of the AIDS Drug Development, Politics & Profits.* New York: HarperCollins.

Associated Press (1990, August 8). "3rd Suit Against Lilly Antidepressant Drug." *Chicago Tribune.*

Associated Press (1991, January 30). "Shannon Widow Sues Drug Company." *Variety.*

Associated Press Release, San Francisco (1991, November 8). "Daughter Arrested in 'Cannibal' Attack."

Associated Press (1992, February 13). "FDA Strips Breast Implant Critic of His Role." *Washington Post,* p. A24.

Associated Press (1992, October 12). "White House Plan Bodes Ill for Drug Safety, Report Says." *Fort Wayne Journal-Gazette,* p. 6A.

Avery, David, and George Winokur (1978, June). "Suicide, Attempted Suicide, and Relapse Rates in Depression." *Archives of General Psychiatry* 35:749–753.

Avorn, Jerry, Milton Chen, and Robert Hartley (1982, July). "Scientific versus Commercial Sources of Influence on the Prescribing Behavior of Physicians." *American Journal of Medicine* 73:5–28.

Baghurst, Peter A., Anthony J. McMichael, Neil R. Wiggs, Graham V. Vimpani, Evelyn F. Robertson, Russell J. Roberts, and Shi-Lu Tong (1992, October 29). "Environmental Exposure to Lead and Children's Intelligence at the Age of Seven Years." *New England Journal of Medicine* 327:1279–1284.

Baird, R. E. (1991, December 13). "Embattled Drug at Issue in Death." *Colorado Daily* (University of Colorado).

Baker, Barbara (1993, July). "Limited Data Suggest Fluoxetine Safe for Children." *Clinical Psychiatry News,* p. 18.

Baldessarini, Ross J., and Elda Marsh (1990, February). "Fluoxetine and Side Effects." *Archives of General Psychiatry* 47: 191–192.

Balter, M. B., and J. Levin (1969). "The Nature and Extent of Psychotropic Drug Usage in the United States." *Psychopharmacology Bulletin* 5:3.

Bargmann, Eve, Sidney M. Wolfe, Joan Levin and the Public Citizen Health Research Group (1983). *Stopping Valium.* New York: Warner Books.

Barinaga, Marcia (1994, March 4). "How the Brain Weeds Its Garden." *Science* 263:1225.

Baron, Bruce M., Ann-Marie Odgen, Barry W. Siegel, James Stegeman, Richard C. Ursillo, and Mark W. Dudley (1988). "Rapid Down Regulation of B [editor, beta]-adrenoreceptors by Coadministration of Desipramine and Fluoxetine." *European Journal of Pharmacology* 154:125–134.

Belles, Christopher (1993, November 8). "Happiness in a Pill." *The Eagle* (American University, Washington, D.C.), p. B1.

Belli, Anne (1991, June 23). "Family Takes on Drug Firm: Prozac Blamed in Man's Suicide." *The Dallas Morning News.*

Bergstromm, Richard F., Albert L. Peyton, and Louis Lemberger (1992). "Quantification and Mechanism of Fluoxetine and Tricyclic Antidepressant Interaction." *Clinical Pharmacology and Therapeutics* 51:239–248.

Berry, Wendell (1977). *The Unsettling of America; Culture & Agriculture.* San Francisco: Sierra Club Books.

Blier, Pierre, and Claude de Montigny (1983, June). "Electrophysiological Investigations on the Effect of Repeated Zimelidine Administration on Serotonergic Neurotransmission in the Rat." *Journal of Neuroscience* 3:1270–1278.

Blier, Pierre, Yves Chaput, and Claude de Montigny (1988). "Long-term 5-HT Reuptake Blockade, But No Monoamine Oxidase Inhibition, Decreases the Function of Terminal 5-HT Autoreceptors; an Electrophysiological Study of the Rat Brain." *Naunyn-Schmiederberg's Archives of Pharmacology* 337:246–254.

Blodgett, Nancy (1990, November). "Eli Lilly Drug Targeted." *ABA Journal,* p. 28.

Bost, Robert O., and Philip M. Kemp (1992, March/April). "A Possible Association Between Fluoxetine Use and Suicide." *Journal of Analytical Toxicology* 16:142–145.

Boulos, C., S. Kutcher, D. Gardner, and E. Young (1992). "An Open Naturalistic Trial of Fluoxetine in Adolescents and Young Adults with Treatment-Resistant Major Depression." *Journal of Child and Adolescent Psychopharmacology* 2:103–111.

Bower, Bruce (1992, October 10). "Efficacy of Antidepressants Challenged." *Science* 142:231.

Boyer, W. F., and J. P. Feighner (1992, February). "An Overview of Paroxetine." *Journal of Clinical Psychiatry* 53:Supplement, pp. 3–6.

Brandes, Lorne J., Randi J. Arron, R. Patricia Bogdanovic, Jiangang Tong, Cheryl L. F. Zaborniak, Georgina R. Hogg, Robert C. Warrington, Wei Fang, and Frank S. LaBella (1992, July 1). "Stimulation of Malignant Growth in Rodents by Antidepressant Drugs at Clinically Relevant Doses." *Cancer Research* 52:3796–3800.

Brandt, Aviva L. (1994, March 3). "Doctor Advises Reporter to Check Out Prozac." Associated Press wire service.

Brandt, Aviva L. (1994, March 4). "'Piper' Suggests Side Dish at Meal with Writer: Prozac." *The Arizona Republic,* p. 1.

Brataas, Anne (1991, March 10). "Light in the Darkness." *St. Paul Pioneer Press,* p. 1F.

Breggin, Ginger, and Peter Breggin (1992, spring). "Feminist Paradigms and Conflict Resolution." *ICAR Newsletter* (Institute for Conflict Analysis and Resolution, George Mason University), p. 1.

Breggin, Peter (1971). *The Crazy from the Sane* (a novel). New York: Lyle Stuart.

Breggin, Peter (1979). *Electroshock: Its Brain-Disabling Effects.* New York: Springer Publishing Company.

Breggin, Peter (1980). "Brain-Disabling Therapies." In Valenstein, E. (ed.): *The Psychosurgery Debate.* San Francisco, W. H. Freeman.

Breggin, Peter (1981a). "Disabling the Brain with Electroshock." In Dongier, M., and E. D. Wittkower (eds.): *Divergent Views in Psychiatry.* Hagerstown, Maryland: Harper & Row.

Breggin, Peter (1981b). "Psychosurgery as Brain-Disabling Therapy." In Dongier, M. and E. D. Wittkower (eds.): *Di-*

vergent Views in Psychiatry. Hagerstown, Maryland: Harper & Row.

Breggin, Peter (1983a) *Psychiatric Drugs: Hazards to the Brain.* New York: Springer Publishing Company.

Breggin, Peter (1983b). "Iatrogenic Helplessness in Authoritarian Psychiatry." In Morgan, R. F. (ed.): *The Iatrogenics Handbook.* Toronto: IPI Publishing Company.

Breggin, Peter (1990a): "Brain Damage, Dementia and Persistent Cognitive Dysfunction Associated with Neuroleptic Drugs: Evidence, Etiology, Implications." *Journal of Mind Behavior* 11:425–464.

Breggin, Peter (1990b, March). "The Scapegoating of American Children." *The Rights Tenet* [newsletter of the National Association for Rights Protection and Advocacy], p. 3. Reprinted from the *Wall Street Journal,* November 7, 1989, p. A30.

Breggin, Peter (1991a). *Toxic Psychiatry: Why Therapy, Empathy and Love Must Replace the Drugs, Electroshock and Biochemical Theories of the "New Psychiatry."* New York: St. Martin's Press.

Breggin, Peter (1992a) *Beyond Conflict: From Self-Help and Psychotherapy to Peacemaking.* New York: St. Martin's Press.

Breggin, Peter (1992b, summer). "News and Views on Psychiatry: The Violence Initiative—A Racist Biomedical Program for Social Control." *The Rights Tenet,* pp. 3–8.

Breggin, Peter (1992c, September 18). "U.S. Hasn't Given Up Linking Genes to Crime." *New York Times,* p. A34.

Breggin, Peter (1992d, September 23). "Report from the Center for the Study of Psychiatry: The Federal Violence Initiative." Bethesda, Maryland: Center for the Study of Psychiatry.

Breggin, Peter (1992e). "A Case of Fluoxetine-Induced Stimulant Side Effects with Suicidal Ideation Associated with a Possible Withdrawal Reaction ('Crashing')." *International Journal of Risk and Safety in Medicine* 3:325–328.

Breggin, Peter (1992f, March). "The Return of ECT." *Readings: A Journal of Reviews and Commentary in Mental Health* 7: No. 1, pp. 12–17.

Breggin, Peter (1992g, February 11). "The President's Sleeping Pill and Its Makers." *New York Times,* p. A18.

Breggin, Peter (1992h, Winter/Spring). "News and Views on Psychiatry: Prozac, Suicide and Violence: An Analysis with Reports from the Prozac Survivors Support Group, Inc." *The Rights Tenet,* pp. 4–6.

Breggin, Peter (1993a). "News and Views on Psychiatry: The FDA—More Harm Than Good?" *The Rights Tenet,* pp. 3–5.

Breggin, Peter (1993b). "Psychiatry's Role in the Holocaust." *International Journal of Risk and Safety in Medicine* 4:133–148.

Breggin, Peter (1993c). "Parallels between Neuroleptic Effects and Lethargic Encephalitis: The Production of Dyskinesias and Cognitive Disorders." *Brain and Cognition* 23:8–27.

Breggin, Peter, and Ginger Breggin (1993a, March). "A Biomedical Programme for Urban Violence Control in the US: The Dangers of Psychiatric Social Control." *Changes: An International Journal of Psychology and Psychotherapy* 11: No. 1, pp. 59–71.

Breggin, Peter, and Ginger Breggin (1993b, April). "The Federal Violence Initiative: Threats to Black Children (And Others)." *Psych Discourse* [journal of the Association of Black Psychologists] 24: No. 4, pp. 8–11.

Breggin, Peter, and Ginger Breggin (1994, in press for the fall). *The War Against Children.* New York: St. Martin's Press.

Brewerton, Timothy D. (1991). "Fluoxetine-Induced Suicidality, Serotonin, and Seasonality." *Biological Psychiatry* 30:190–196.

British Medical Association and Royal Pharmaceutical Society of Great Britain (1991, September). *British National Formulary (BNF).* London, England: The Pharmaceutical Press.

Brown, Gerald L., and Markku I. Linnoila (1990, April). "CSF Serotonin Metabolite (5-HIAA) Studies in Depression, Impulsivity, and Violence." *Journal of Clinical Psychiatry* 51 (supplement), No. 4:31–41.

Brown, Serena-Lynn, and Herman M. van Praag (eds.) (1991). *The Role of Serotonin in Psychiatric Disorders.* New York: Brunner/Mazel.

Bunch, Michael, and Jim Trotter (1991, April 18). "2 Now Dead in Domestic Tragedy; Daughter, a Witness, Traumatized." *The San Diego Union,* p. B1.

Burns, Matthew (1991, December 10). "Pelzer Man Gets 30 Years in Estranged Wife's Slaying." *Greenville Daily* (South Carolina).

Burton, Thomas (1993, February 22). "Eli Lilly & Company Is Scrutinized by Grand Jury." *Wall Street Journal,* p. B-4.

Bymaster, Franklin P., and David T. Wong (1974, August 20). "Effect of Lilly 110140, 3-(p-trifluoromethylphenoxy)-N-methyl-3-tryptophan in Rat Brain." *The Pharmacologist* 16: 302.

Canadian Pharmaceutical Association (1993). *CPS: Compendium of Pharmaceuticals and Specialties.* Ottawa, Ontario: Canadian Pharmaceutical Association.

Candisky, Catherine (1992, October 28). "Son Given 20 Years to Life in Beating Death of Mother." *The Columbus Dispatch* (Ohio).

Carlson, Elliot (1992, July/August). "Critics See FDA Flip-Flop." *AARP Bulletin*, p. 1.

Carrie, Sylvester E., and Markus J. P. Kruesi (1994, February). "Child and Adolescent Psychopharmacology: Progress and Pitfalls." *Psychiatric Annals* 24:83–90.

Cassada, Mary Eva (1991, September 17). "Prozac Noted by Massey's Attorney." *Danville Register & Bee* (Danville, Virginia).

Cassano, Dennis (1991, February 2). "Douglas Simmons Found Dead in His Car." *Star Tribune* (Minneapolis), p. 1B.

Charles, Henrietta (1991, April 20). "Woman Who Took Prozac, Killed Husband Gets Probation." *Press-Telegram* (Long Beach, California).

Chouinard, Guy, and Warren Steiner (1986, May). "A Case of Mania Induced by High-Dose Fluoxetine Treatment." *American Journal of Psychiatry* 143:686.

Cincinnati Enquirer, The (1991, August 28). "Drug Prozac Cited in Murder-for-Hire Case."

Clemens, James A., Barry D. Sawyer, and Benito Cerimele (1977). "Further Evidence That Serotonin Is a Neurotransmitter Involved in the Control of Prolactin Secretion." *Endocrinology* 100:692–698.

Cockburn, Alexander (1992, December 7). "Paradigms of Power: The Case of Eli Lilly." *The Nation*, p. 690.

Cockburn, Alexander (1994, January 31). "Beat the Devil: The Second Great Depression." *The Nation*, p. 116.

Cohn, J. B., and Charles Wilcox (1985, March). "A Comparison of Fluoxetine, Imipramine, and Placebo in Patients with Major Depressive Disorder." *Journal of Clinical Psychiatry* 46 [3, sec.] 2:26–31.

Cole, Jonathan O. (1972). "Clinical Uses of Amphetamines." In Ellinwood, Everett H., Jr., and Sidney Cohen (eds.): *Current Concepts on Amphetamine Abuse.* Rockville, Maryland: National Institute of Mental Health. DHEW Publication No. (HMS) 72–9085. Chapter 16, pp. 163–169.

Connell, P. H. (1966). "Clinical Manifestations and Treatment of Amphetamine Type of Dependence." *Journal of the American Medical Association* 196:718–723.

Consumers Union Report (1972). *Licit and Illicit Drugs* Boston: Little, Brown and Company.

The Courier-Journal (1990, November 3). "Louisville Woman Sues Lilly, Claiming Prozac Made Her Attempt Suicide."

Cowley, Geoffrey (1990, March 26). "The Promise of Prozac." *Newsweek,* pp. 39–41.

Cowley, Geoffrey (1994, February 7). "The Culture of Prozac." *Newsweek,* p. 41–42.

Creaney, W., I. Murray, and D. Healy (1991). "Antidepressant-Induced Suicidal Ideation." *Human Psychopharmacology* 6: 329–332.

Crowner, Martha L., Richard Douyon, Antonio Convit, Pedro Gaztanaga, Jan Volavka, and Robert Bakall (1990). "Akathisia and Violence." *Psychopharmacology Bulletin* 26:115–117.

Daily Courier (West Canada) (1991, April 30). "Man Says New Drug Caused His Actions."

Dasgupta, Krishna (1990, November). "Additional Cases of Suicidal Ideation Associated with Fluoxetine." *American Journal of Psychiatry* 147:1570.

Davila, Edward (1994, March 5). Telephone interview with Peter Breggin concerning Eli Lilly's support of the prosecution in the case against Dwight Harlor, III.

De Cicco, Tony (1984, November 13). Minutes of the "In-House Meeting on Fluoxetine" of the Food and Drug Administration. Present at the meeting were P. Leber, M.D.; T. Hayes, M.D.; H. Lee, Ph.D.; T. Laughren, M.D.; R. Kapit, M.D.; G. Chi, Ph.D.; and T. De Cicco, CSO. Obtained through the Freedom of Information Act.

De Montigny, Claude, Yves Chaput, and Pierre Blier (1990, December). "Modification of Serotonergic Neuron Properties by Long-Term Treatment with Serotonin Reuptake Blockers." *Journal of Clinical Psychiatry* 51:12 (supplement B), pp. 4–9.

Dewan, Mantosh J., and Prakash Masand (1991). "Prozac and Suicide." *Journal of Family Practice* 33:312.

Drake, Robert E., and Ehrlich, Joshua (1985, April). "Suicide Attempts Associated with Akathisia." *American Journal of Psychiatry* 142:499–501.

Duggan, Paul (1991, May 22). "Md. Woman's Lawyer Eyes Insanity Defense Based on Prozac Use." *Washington Post,* p. 1.

DuPont, Robert L. (1993, October 7). "Dear Doctor" letter, accompanied by a two-page publication, "Clinical Trials Today," edited by Elizabeth DuPont Spencer (Fall, 1993). Rockville, Maryland: Institute for Behavior and Health, Inc.

Duran, Marlys (1992, January 10). "Unarmed Bank Robber Gets Probation." *Rocky Mountain News* (Denver, Colorado).

Eagen, Timothy (1994, January 30). "A Washington City Full of Prozac." *New York Times,* p. 16.

Economist, The (London) (1991, January 19). "Prozac and Suicide: Open Verdict," p. 76.

Eddy, Mark, and Steve Lipsher (1991, September 19). "Slay Suspect Mentally Ill: Man Treated with Prozac." *The Denver Post,* p. 1A.

Editorial (1990, August 11). "5-HT Blockers and All That." *Lancet* 336:345–346.

Eli Lilly and Company (1992). "Form 10-K. Annual Report Pursuant to the Section 13 or 15(d) of the Securities and Exchange Act of 1934." For the fiscal year ended December 31, 1992. Washington, D.C.: Securities and Exchange Commission.

Ellinwood, E. H., Jr. (1971). "Assault and Homicide Associated with Amphetamine Abuse." *American Journal of Psychiatry* 120:90.

Ellinwood, E. H., Jr. (1972). "Amphetamine Psychosis: Individuals, Settings, and Sequences." In Ellinwood, Everett H., Jr., and Sidney Cohen (eds.): *Current Concepts on Amphetamine Abuse.* Rockville, Maryland: National Institute of Mental Health. DHEW Publication No. (HMS) 72-9085. Chapter 14, pp. 143–157.

Eppsteiner, Fred (ed.) (1988). *The Paths of Compassion: Writings on Socially Engaged Buddhism.* Berkeley, California: Parallax Press.

Fava, Maurizio, and Jerrold F. Rosenbaum (1990, May). "Suicidality and Fluoxetine: Is There a Relationship." New Research Abstract #475. Presented at the annual meeting of the American Psychiatric Association, New York.

Fava, Maurizio, and Jerrold F. Rosenbaum (1990, July). " 'Anger Attacks': Possible Variants of Panic and Major Depressive Disorders." *American Journal of Psychiatry* 147:867–870.

Fava, Maurizio, and Jerrold F. Rosenbaum (1991, March). "Suicidality and Fluoxetine: Is There Relationship." *Journal of Clinical Psychiatry* 52:108–111.

Fawcett, Jan (1990, November). "Targeting Treatment in Patients with Mixed Symptoms of Anxiety and Depression." *Journal of Clinical Psychiatry* 51:11 (suppl).

Fetner, Harriet, Hazel Watts, and Barbara Geller (1991, September). "Fluoxetine and Preoccupation with Suicide." *American Journal of Psychiatry* 148:258.

Fieve, Ronald R. (1994). *Prozac: Questions and Answers for Patients, Family, and Physicians.* New York: Avon.

Fisher, Seymour, Stephen G. Bryant, and Thomas A. Kent (1993). "Postmarketing Surveillance by Patient Self-monitoring: Trazodone versus Fluoxetine." *Journal of Clinical Psychopharmacology* 13:235–242.

Fisher, Seymour, and Roger Greenberg (1993). "How Sound Is the Double-Blind Desire for Evaluating Drugs?" *Journal of Nervous and Mental Disease* 181:345–350.

Fisher, Seymour, and Roger Greenberg (eds.) (1989). *The Limits of Biological Treatments for Psychological Distress: Comparisons with Psychotherapy and Placebo.* Hillsdale, New Jersey: Lawrence Erlbaum.

Fishman, Howard (ed.) (1990, October, Supplement). "Clinical Issues on Treatment-Resistant Depression [report on a presentation by David L. Dunner]." *Psychiatric Times.*

Food and Drug Administration (1985, January 31). "Psychopharmacology Drugs Advisory Committee. (Workshop) Twenty-seventh Meeting." Department of Health and Human Services, Public Health Service, Food and Drug Administration, Rockville, Maryland. Obtained through the Freedom of Information Act.

Food and Drug Administration (1985, March 28). "Review and Evaluation of Efficacy Data." NDA 18-936 (Prozac). Internal document of the Department of Health and Human Services, Public Health Service, Food and Drug Administration, Center for Drug Evaluation and Research. Obtained through the Freedom of Information Act.

Food and Drug Administration (1985, December 30). "Review and Evaluation of Clinical Data. Amendment." NDA 18-936 (Prozac). Internal document of the Department of Health and Human Services, Public Health Service, Food and Drug Administration, Center for Drug Evaluation and Research. Obtained through the Freedom of Information Act.

Food and Drug Administration (1988, October 3). "Summary Basis of Approval [SBA]." NDA 18-936 (Prozac). Internal document of the Department of Health and Human Services, Public Health Service, Food and Drug Administration, Center for Drug Evaluation and Research. Obtained through the Freedom of Information Act.

Food and Drug Administration (1991, September 12). "Participation of James L. Claghorn, M.D., as a Member of FDA's Psychopharmacologic Drugs Advisory Committee. Memorandum for the Public Record." Department of Health and Human Services, Public Health Service, Food and Drug Administration. Rockville, Maryland. Obtained through the Freedom of Information Act.

Food and Drug Administration (1991, September 13). "Participation of Jeffrey A. Lieberman, M.D., as a Member of FDA's Psychopharmacologic Drugs Advisory Committee. Memorandum for the Public Record." Department of Health and Human Services, Public Health Service, Food and Drug Administration. Rockville, Maryland. Obtained through the Freedom of Information Act.

Food and Drug Administration (1991, September 16). "Participation of David L. Dunner, M.D., as a member of FDA's Psychopharmacologic Drugs Advisory Committee. Memorandum for the Public Record." Department of Health and Human Services, Public Health Service, Food and Drug Administration, Rockville, Maryland. Obtained through the Freedom of Information Act.

Food and Drug Administration (1991, September 17). "Participation of Michael E. Stanley, Ph.D., as a consultant to FDA's Center for Drug Evaluation and Research. Memorandum for the Public Record." Department of Health and Human Services, Public Health Service, Food and Drug Administration. Rockville, Maryland. Obtained through the Freedom of Information Act.

Food and Drug Administration (1991, September 20a). "Psychopharmacology Drugs Advisory Committee. Thirty-fourth Meeting." Department of Health and Human Services, Public Health Service, Food and Drug Administration, Rockville, Maryland. Obtained through the Freedom of Information Act.

Food and Drug Administration (1991, September 20b). "Conflict of Interest Statement for the Psychopharmacologic Drugs

Advisory Committee." Department of Health and Human Services, Public Health Service, Food and Drug Administration, Rockville, Maryland. Obtained through the Freedom of Information Act.

Fossey, Dian (1983). *Gorillas in the Mist.* New York: Houghton Mifflin Company.

Foundation for Advanced Education in the Sciences (FAES) (1993). "President's Report by Karl A. Piez, Ph.D." *Annual Report.*

Frances, R. J., and John E. Franklin (1988). "Alcohol and Other Psychoactive Substance Use Disorders." In Talbott, John A., Robert E. Hales, and Stuart C. Yudofsky (eds.): *Textbook of Psychiatry.* Washington, D.C.: American Psychiatric Press, 1988. Chapter 11, pp. 313–355.

Freudenheim, Milt (1990, July 17). "More Gilding for Lilly as a New Drug Stars." *New York Times,* p. D1.

Fudge, J. L., P. J. Perry, M. J. Garvey, and M. W. Kelly (1990). "A Comparison of the Effect of Fluoxetine and Trazodone on the Cognitive Functioning of Depressed Outpatients." *Journal of Affective Disorders* 18:275–280.

Fuller, Ray W. (1986). "Biochemical Pharmacology of the Serotonin System." *Advances in Neurology* 43:469–480.

Fuller, Ray W. (1992, January 7). Letter to Peter Breggin concerning Breggin's discussion of serotonergic mechanisms in *Toxic Psychiatry.* Indianapolis, Indiana, Lilly Research Labs.

Fuller, Ray W., and Charles M. Beasley (1991, September). "Fluoxetine Mechanism of Action." *Journal of the American Academy of Child and Adolescent Psychiatry* 30:849.

Fuller, Ray W., Kenneth W. Perry, and Bryan B. Molloy (1974). "Effect of an Uptake Inhibitor on Serotonin Metabolism in Rat Brain." *Life Sciences* 15:1161–1171.

Fuller, Ray W., and David T. Wong (1977, July). "Inhibition of Serotonin Reuptake." *Federation Proceedings* 36:2154–2158.

Gardner, Fred (1994, February 23). "Notes from the City: Prozac 'Abuse' Interview with Darryl Inaba." *Anderson Valley Advertiser* (Boonville, California), p. 5.

Gawin, Frank H., and Everett H. Ellinwood, Jr. (1989). "Stimulants." In *Treatments of Psychiatric Disorders: A Task Force Report of the American Psychiatric Association.* Washington, D.C.: American Psychiatric Association. Chapter 130, pp. 1218–1240.

Gilman, Alfred Goodman, Theodore W. Rall, Alan S. Nies, and

Palmer Taylor (eds.) (1991). *The Pharmacological Basis of Therapeutic, VIII.* New York: Pergamon Press.

Gold, Mark S., and Michael H. Kronig (1984). "Comprehensive Thyroid Evaluation in Psychiatric Patients." In Hall, R. C. W., and R. P. Beresford (eds.). *Handbook of Diagnostic Psychiatric Procedures, Volume I.* Jamaica, New York: Spectrum Publications, Inc., 1984. Chapter 2, pp. 29–45.

Goldman, Marcus J., Lester Grinspoon, Susan Hunter-Jones (1990, October). "Ritualistic Use of Fluoxetine by a Former Substance Abuser." *American Journal of Psychiatry* 147:1377.

Goodall, Jane (1986). *The Chimpanzees of Gombe: Patterns of Behavior.* Cambridge, Massachusetts: Belknap Press of Harvard University Press.

Gorman, Jack M., Michael R. Liebowitz, Abby J. Fyer, Deborah Goetz, Raphael B. Campeas, Minna R. Fyer, Sharon O. Davies, and Donald F. Klein (1987, October). "An Open Trial of Fluoxetine in the Treatment of Panic Attacks." *Journal of Clinical Psychopharmacology* 5:329–332.

Graedon, Joe, and Teresa Graedon (1990, August 10). "Is the Cure Causing the Disease." *The State Journal* (Frankfort, Kentucky), p. A6.

Graedon, Joe, and Teresa Graedon (1991, April 22). "The People's Pharmacy: Did Prozac Drive Daughter to Suicide?" Syndicated King Features Column, 235 East 45th Street, New York, NY 10017.

Greenberg, Roger P., and Seymour Fisher (1989). "Examining Antidepressant Effectiveness: Findings, Ambiguities, and Some Vexing Puzzles." In Fisher, Seymour, and Roger P. Greenberg (eds.). *The Limits of Biological Treatments for Psychological Distress.* Hillsdale, New Jersey: Erlbaum, pp. 1–37.

Greenberg, Roger P., Robert F. Bornstein, Michael D. Greenberg, and Seymour Fisher (1992). "A Meta-analysis of Antidepressant Outcome Under 'Blinder' Conditions." *Journal of Consulting and Clinical Psychology* 60:664–669.

Grinspoon, Lester, and James Bakalar (1976). *Cocaine.* New York: Basic Books.

Grinspoon, Lester, and James Bakalar (1985). "Drug Dependence: Nonnarcotic Agents." In Kaplan, Harold I., and Benjamin J. Sadock (eds.). *Comprehensive Textbook of Psychiatry.* Baltimore: Williams & Wilkins. Chapter 22.2, pp. 1003–1015.

Grinspoon, Lester, and Peter Hedblom (1975). *The Speed Cul-*

ture: *Amphetamine Use and Abuse in America*. Cambridge, Massachusetts: Harvard University Press.

Gualtieri, C. Thomas (1991, December). "Paradoxical Effects of Fluoxetine." *Journal of Clinical Psychopharmacology* 11:393–394.

Gualtieri, C. Thomas, and Robert Sovner (1989, December). "Akathisia and Tardive Akathisia." *Psychiatric Aspects of Mental Retardation Reviews*. 8: No. 12, pp. 83–87.

Gubin, S. (1993, March). "Prozac: The Miracle Drug?" *Sojourner*, pp. 5H–6H.

Guttman, E. (1939). "Discussion of Benzedrine; Uses and Abuses." *Proclamations of the Royal Society of Medicine* 32: 388.

Hersh, Carol B., Mae S. Sokol, and Cynthia R. Pfeffer (1991, September). "Transient Psychosis with Fluoxetine." *Journal of the Academy of Child and Adolescent Psychiatry* 30:851.

Higham, Scott (1991, September 7). "Kathy Willets: Prozac Drug Made Me Insatiable." *Miami Herald* (Florida).

Higley, J., P. Mehlman, D. Taub, S. Higley, S. Suomi, M. Linnoila, and J.Vickers (1992). "Cerebrospinal Fluid Monoamine and Adrenal Correlates of Aggression in Free-ranging Rhesus Monkeys." *Archives of General Psychiatry* 49:436–441.

Higley, J., W. Thompson, M. Champoux, D. Goldman, M. Hasert, G. Kraemer, J. Scanlan, S. Suomi, and M. Linnoila (1993, August). "Paternal and Maternal Genetic and Environmental Contributions to Cerebrospinal Fluid Monoamine Metabolites in Rhesus Monkeys (Macaca mulatta)." *Archives of General Psychiatry* 50:615–623.

Hilgers, DeAnne (1991, November 20). "Attempted Murder Charge Filed." *Forum* (Fargo, North Dakota).

Hilts, Philip J. (1993, December 10). "Early Unreported Illnesses Linked to Deadly Drug." *New York Times*, p. A22.

Hinmon, Derrick, and Kathy Scruggs (1991, August 23). "Nashville Man Charged in Midtown Fire." *The Atlanta Journal* (Georgia).

Hoehn-Saric, Rudolf, John R. Lipsey, and Daniel R. McLeod (1990, October). "Apathy and Indifference in Patients on Fluvoxamine and Fluoxetine." *Journal of Clinical Psychopharmacology* 10:343–345.

Hoffman, Brian B., and Robert J. Lefkowitz (1991). "Catecholamines and Sympathomimetic Drugs." In Gilman, Alfred Goodman, Theodore W. Rall, Alan S. Nies, and Palmer Taylor (eds.): *The Pharmacological Basis of Therapeutics.* New York: Pergamon Press. Chapter 10, pp. 187–220.

Hooper, L. (1992, October 13). "Study Shows Long-Term Care To Be More Effective in Treating Depression." *Wall Street Journal,* p. B7.

Hoover, Cynthia E. (1990, November). "Additional Cases of Suicidal Ideation Associated with Fluoxetine." *American Journal of Psychiatry* 147:1570–1571.

Hoover, Cynthia E. (1991, April). "Suicidal Ideation Not Associated with Fluoxetine." *American Journal of Psychiatry* 148:543.

Hughes, Richard, and Robert Brewin (1979). *The Tranquilizing of America.* New York: Harcourt Brace Jovanovich, Inc.

Humphries, John E., Munsey S. Wheby, and Scott R. Vandenberg (1990, July). "Fluoxetine and Bleeding Time." *Archives of Pathology and Laboratory Medicine* 114:727–728.

Hunt, Liz, and Glenn Frankel (1991, October 3). "Britain Takes Halcion Sleeping Pills Off Market." *Washington Post,* p. A3.

Inquisition into the death of Richard Barger, who met his death on September 14, 1989 (and eight others, including Joseph Wesbecker, who died of suicide) (1989, November 22). Dr. Richard Greathouse, Jefferson County Coroner, Kentucky.

Jaffe, Jerome H. (1989). "Drug Dependence: Opioids, Nonnarcotics, Nicotine (Tobacco) and Caffeine." In Kaplan, Harold I., and Benjamin J. Sadock (eds.): *Comprehensive Textbook of Psychiatry, V.* Chapter 13.1, pp. 642–686. Baltimore: Williams & Wilkins.

Jafri, Alima B., and William M. Greenberg (1991, September). "Fluoxetine Side Effects." *Journal of the American Academy of Child and Adolescent Psychiatry* 30:852.

Jain, J., B. Birmaher, M. Garcia, M. Al-Shabbout, and N. Ryan (1992). "Fluoxetine in Children and Adolescents with Mood Disorders: A Chart Review of Efficacy and Adverse Reactions." *Journal of Child and Adolescent Psychopharmacology* 2:259–265.

Jamison, Kay Redfield (1993, August 8). "Tempest in a Capsule." *Washington Post Book World,* p. 2.

Jerome, Laurence (1991, September). "Hypomania with Fluoxetine." *Journal of the American Academy of Child and Adolescent Psychiatry* 30:850–851.

Jonas, Jeffrey M., and Ron Schaumburg (1991). *Everything You Need to Know About Prozac.* New York: Bantam.

Jonas, J. M. (1992, October). Dr. Jeffrey M. Jonas, director of CNS clinical development at Upjohn, replies to Fred Baughman, Jr.. *Clinical Psychiatry News,* p. 5.

Jones, Ernest (1953). *The Life and Work of Sigmund Freud, Volume I.* New York: Basic Books.

Journal of the American Medical Association. (1992, December 23/30). "Vote of Confidence for FDA Advisory Committees, But Conflict of Interest Questions Remain." 268:3417.

Journal of Clinical Psychiatry (1993, December). "Neuroleptic-Induced Deficit Syndrome (SIDS)." 54:493–500.

Kalda, Riho (1993, March). "Media- or Fluoxetine-Induced Akathisia." *American Journal of Psychiatry* 150:531–532.

Kapit, Richard M. [same as R. M. Kapit] (1986, March). "Safety Review of NDA 18-936 [Prozac]." Internal document of the Department of Health and Human Services, Public Health Service, Food and Drug Administration, Center for Drug Evaluation and Research. Obtained through the Freedom of Information Act.

Kapit, R. M. (1986, December 17). "Response to Dr. Laughren's Q's Regarding Review of Safety Update, Memo #3." NDA 18-936. Internal document of the Department of Health and Human Services, Public Health Service, Food and Drug Administration, Center for Drug Evaluation and Research. Obtained through the Freedom of Information Act.

Kapit, R. M. (1988, March 4). "Memorandum: Revision of Clinical Portion of Prozac SBA." NDA 18-936. Internal document, Department of Health and Human Services, Public Health Service, Food and Drug Administration, Center for Drug Evaluation and Research. Obtained through the Freedom of Information Act.

Karel, R. (1991, June 7). "Members React to Campaign Discrediting Prozac, Psychiatry." *Psychiatric News,* p. 18.

Karel, Richard. (1993, January 1). "Halcion Partially Blamed in Homicide Despite FDA Ruling Upholding Data." *Psychiatric News,* p. 4.

Keckich, Walter A. (1978, November 10). "Neuroleptics: Violence as a Manifestation of Akathisia." *Journal of the American Medical Association* 240:2185.

Kelsey, Frances O. (1984, October 26). Letter from Frances Kelsey, Ph.D., M.D., Director of Division of Scientific Investigations, Office of Compliance, Center for Drugs and Biologics, the Food and Drug Administration, to Jay B. Cohn,

M.D., 3505 Long Beach Boulevard, Suite 2-E, Long Beach, California. Obtained through the Freedom of Information Act.

Kelsey, Frances O. (1984, October 26). Letter from Frances Kelsey, Ph.D., M.D., Director of Division of Scientific Investigations, Office of Compliance, Center for Drugs and Biologics, the Food and Drug Administration to Bernard I. Grosser, M.D. Obtained through the Freedom of Information Act.

Kelsey, Frances O. (1984, December 13). Letter from Frances Kelsey, Ph.D., M.D., Director of Division of Scientific Investigations, Office of Compliance, Center for Drugs and Biologics, the Food and Drug Administration to Faruk S. Abuzzahab, Sr., M.D., Ph.D. Obtained through the Freedom of Information Act.

Kifner, John (1990, November 9). "Police Say Kahane Suspect Took Anti-Depression Drugs." *New York Times,* p. B3.

Kilgore, Christine (1991, March). "Psychiatrists Doubt Claims That Prozac Induces Violence." *Clinical Psychiatry News,* Vol. 19, No. 3, p. 1.

King, Robert A., Mark A. Riddle, Phillip B. Chappell, Maureen T. Hardin, George M. Anderson, Paul Lombroso, and Larry Scahill (1991, March). "Emergence of Self-destructive Phenomena in Children and Adolescents During Fluoxetine Treatment." *Journal of the American Academy of Child and Adolescent Psychiatry* 30:179–186.

Kline, Harrison Douglas, *et al.* (plaintiffs) v. The Upjohn Company, Dr. Louis Fabre, *et al.* (defendants.). "Plaintiffs' Original Petition and Jury Demand." Cause No. 93-13277 in the District Court of Dallas County, Texas. December 22, 1993.

Koizumi, Hisako (1991, July). "Fluoxetine and Suicidal Ideation." *Journal of the American Academy of Child and Adolescent Psychiatry* 30:695.

Kolata, Gina (1992, January 26). "Questions Raised on Ability of F.D.A. to Protect Public." *New York Times,* p. 1.

Korn, Martin L., Moshe Kotler, Avi Molcho, Alexander J. Botsis, Daniel Grosz, Clarence Chen, Robert Plutchik, Serena-Lynn Brown, and Herman M. van Pragg (1992). "Suicide and Violence Associated with Panic Attacks." *Biological Psychiatry* 31:607–612.

Kosten, Thomas R. (1993, February). "Pharmacotherapies for Cocaine Abuse." *Psychiatric Times,* p. 25.

Kosterlitz, J. (1987, April 4). "Health Focus: Drugs for Sale." *National Journal*, p. 850.

Kotulak, R. (1993, April 15). "Reshaping Brain for Better Future." *Chicago Tribune*, p. 1.

Kotulak, R. (1993, December 12). "Tracking Down the Monster Within Us." *Chicago Tribune*, p. 1.

Kotulak, R. (1993, December 13). "How Brain Chemistry Unleashes Violence." *Chicago Tribune*, p. 1.

Kotulak, R. (1993, December 14). "Why Some Kids Turn Violent." *Chicago Tribune*, p. 1.

Kotulak, R. (1993, December 15). "New Drugs Break Spell of Violence." *Chicago Tribune*, p. 1.

Kramer, John (1972). "Introduction to Amphetamine Abuse." In Ellinwood, Everett H., Jr. and Sidney Cohen (eds.): *Current Concepts on Amphetamine Abuse.* Rockville, Maryland: National Institute of Mental Health. DHEW Publicaton No. (HMS) 72-9085. Chapter 18, pp. 177–185.

Kramer, Peter (1993). *Listening to Prozac.* New York: Viking.

Kruesi, M., J. Rapoport, S. Hamburger, E. Hibbs, W. Potter, M. Lenane, and G. Brown (1990, May). "Cerebrospinal Fluid Monoamine Metabolites, Aggression, and Impulsivity in Disruptive Behavior Disorders of Children and Adolescents." *Archives of General Psychiatry* 47:419–426.

Kruesi, M., E. Hibbs, T. Zahn, C. Keysor, S. Hamburger, J. Bartko, and J. Rapoport (1992, June). "A 2-Year Prospective Follow-up Study of Children and Adolescents with Disruptive Behavior Disorders: Prediction by Cerebrospinal Fluid 5-Hydroxyindoleacetic Acid, Homovanillic Acid, and Automatic Measures?" *Archives of General Psychiatry* 49:429–435.

Laporta, Marc, Guy Chouinard, David Goldbloom, and Linda Beauclair (1987, November). "Hypomania Induced by Sertraline, a New Serotonin Reuptake Inhibitor." *American Journal of Psychiatry* 144:1513–1514.

Laurence, Leslie (1994, April 20). "Estrogen Used Against Depression." *San Jose Mercury News.*

Leake, Chauncey D. (1971, July 7). "Developer of Amphetamines Reports History of Drug's Use." *Psychiatric News*, p. 5.

Lebegue, Breck (1987, December). "Mania Precipitated by Fluoxetine." *American Journal of Psychiatry* 144:1620.

Leccese, Arthur P., and William H. Lyness (1984). "The Effects of Putative 5-Hydroxytryptamine Receptor Active Agents on

D-amphetamine Self-administration in Controls and Rats with 5,7-Dihydroxytryptamine Median Forebrain Bundle Lesions." *Brain Research* 303:153–162.

Lee, Gary (1993, October 22). "Studies Give Pesticides Role in Breast Cancer." *Washington Post,* p. A20.

Lee, J. Hillary (1985, March 28). See Food and Drug Administration (1985, March 28).

Lee, J. Hillary (1985, December 30). See Food and Drug Administration (1985, December 30).

Lee, J. Hillary (1987, March 12). "Review and Evaluation of Clinical Data." NDA 18-936. Internal document, Department of Health and Human Services, Public Health Service, Food and Drug Administration, Center for Drug Evaluation and Research. Obtained through the Freedom of Information Act.

Lensgraf, S. Jay, and Armando R. Favazza (1990, November). "Antidepressant-Induced Mania." *American Journal of Psychiatry* 147:1569.

Levine, Louise R., Sidney Rosenblatt, and Janet Bosworth (1987). "Use of a Serotonin Re-uptake Inhibitor, Fluoxetine, in the Treatment of Obesity." *International Journal of Obesity* 2 (supplement 3):185–190.

Lewis, Neil (1993, March 7). "Drug Companies Are Fighting Image of Price Gougers." *New York Times,* p. A1.

Lily Deutschland Ltd. (1992, March 16). "Information Concerning Use of Fluctin." Certified translation by Berlitz Translation Center, Woodland Hills, California.

Limbacher, Jolene (1991, January 3). "Drug Gave Me Rage, Wooster Man Says." *Akron Beacon Journal* (Ohio), p. A1.

Lipinski Jr., Joseph F., Gopinath Mallaya, Paula Zimmerman, Harrison G. Pope, Jr. (1989, September). "Fluoxetine-Induced Akathisia: Clinical and Theoretical Implications." *Journal of Clinical Psychiatry* 50:9.

Los Angeles Daily Journal (1990, September 7). "Defense Attorney Says 'Prozac' Made His Client Commit Murder."

Los Angeles Times (1990, August 27). "Prozac in Abbie Hoffman Death?"

Louie, Alan K., Richard A. Lannon, and Luriko J. Ajari (1994, March). "Withdrawal Reaction After Sertraline Discontinuation." *American Journal of Psychiatry* 151:450–451.

Lyness, W. H. (1983). "Effect of L-tryptophan Pretreatment on D-amphetamine Self-administration." *Substance and Alcohol Actions/Misuse* 4:305–312.

Lyness, W. H., N. M. Friedle, and K. E. Moore (1980). "Increased Self-administration of D-amphetamine After Destruction of 5-Hydroxytryptaminergic Neurons." *Pharmacology Biochemistry & Behavior* 22:937–941.

Mandalos, George E. and Bonnie L. Szarek (1990). "Dose-Related Paranoid Reaction Associated with Fluoxetine." *Journal of Nervous and Mental Disease* 178:57–58.

Manders, Dean W. (1992, October). "The Curious Continuing Ban of L-Tryptophan." *Townsend Letter for Doctors*, p. 880.

Mann, J. John, and Shitij Kapur (1991, November). "The Emergence of Suicidal Ideation and Behavior During Antidepressant Pharmacology." *Archives of General Psychiatry* 48:1027–1033.

Marcus, Amy Dockser (1991, February 7). "Murder Trials Introduce Prozac Defense." *Wall Street Journal*, p. B9.

Marcus, Amy Dockser (1991, April 9). "Prozac Firm Fights Drug's Use As Defense." *Wall Street Journal*, p. B8.

Marcus, Amy Dockser, and Wade Lambert (1991, June 6). "Eli Lilly to Pay." *Wall Street Journal*.

Masand, Prakash, Sanjay Gupta, and Mantosh Dewan (1991, February 7). "Suicidal Ideation Related to Fluoxetine Treatment." *New England Journal of Medicine* 324:420.

Maxmen, Jerrold S. (1991). *Psychotropic Drugs Fast Facts*. New York: W. W. Norton.

McKenna, Terence (1992). *Food of the Gods: The Search for the Original Tree of Knowledge—A Radical History of Plants, Drugs, and Human Evolution*. New York: Bantam Books.

McLaughlin, Craig (1990, May 16). "The Perils of Prozac." *San Francisco Bay Guardian*, p. 17.

The Medical Letter: On Drugs and Therapeutics. (1990, September 7). "Fluoxetine (Prozac) Revisited." 32(826):83–85.

Melillo, W. (1993, June 11). "Britain Denies Upjohn Approval for Halcion: 'Concern Must Be for Patients,' Official Says." *Washington Post*, p. A3.

Meltzer, H. Y., M. Young, J. Metz, V. S. Fang, P. M. Schyve, and R. C. Arora (1979). "Extrapyramidal Side Effects and Increased Serum Prolactin Following Fluoxetine, a New Antidepressant." *Journal of Neural Transmission* 45:165–175.

Miller, Alice (1990). *Banished Knowledge: Facing Childhood Injuries*. New York: Anchor Books.

Miller, Michael (1994, March 31). "Listening to Eli Lilly: Prozac Hysteria Has Gone Too Far." *Wall Street Journal*, p. B1.

Miller, Richard A. (1990, November). "Discussion of Fluoxetine and Suicidal Tendencies." *American Journal of Psychiatry* 147:1571.

Mintz, Morton (1965). *The Therapeutic Nightmare.* New York: Houghton Mifflin Company.

Mooty, Melinda (1991, July 4). "Valley Woman's Lawsuit Links Drug to Suicide Attempt." *The Arizona Republic.*

Muijen, M., D. Roy, T. Silverstone, A. Mehmet, and M. Christie (1988). "A Comparative Clinical Trial of Fluoxetine, Mianserin and Placebo in Depressed Patients." *Acta Psychiatrica Scandinavica* 78:384–390.

Murray, Michael J., and Daniel Hooberman (1993, January). "Fluoxetine and Prolonged Erection." *American Journal of Psychiatry* 150:167–168.

Myers, R. D., and W. L. Veale (1968). "Alcohol Preference in the Rat: Reduction Following Depletion of Brain Serotonin." *Science New York* 160:1469–1471.

Nash, J. Frank, and Herbert Y. Meltzer (1991). "Neuroendocrine Studies in Psychiatric Disorders: The Role of Serotonin." In Brown, Serena-Lynn, and Herman M. van Praag (eds.): *The Role of Serotonin in Psychiatric Disorders.* New York: Brunner/Mazel. Chapter 4, pp. 57–90.

Nathanson, Larry (1990, July 15). "Eli Lilly Sued for $150M Over 'Wonder Drug.' " *New York Post.*

National Institute of Drug Abuse (1989). "National Household Survey on Drug Abuse: Population Estimates 1988." Rockville, Maryland: NIDA.

News & Record (Halifax, Virginia). (1991, April 29). "Moneymaker Appeals for Prozac Info," p. 1.

Newsweek (1990, March 26). "Prozac: A Breakthrough Drug for Depression," p. 38.

Newsweek (1994, February 7). "Beyond Prozac," p. 36.

Novelli, Barbara J., individually; Donna Wartenberg, appointed next friend and guardian, plaintiff, v. The State of Alaska, *et al.,* defendants. In the Superior Court for the State of Alaska, Third Judicial District at Anchorage, Case No. 3AN-89-333 Civil. The case was tried in 1991.

Office of Inspector General, Richard P. Kusserow, Inspector General (1992, June). *Prescription Drug Advertisements in Medical Journals.* Rockville, Maryland: Department of Health and Human Services. OEI-01-90-00482.

Papp, Laszlo A., and Jack M. Gorman (1990, October). "Suicidal Preoccupation During Fluoxetine Treatment." *American Journal of Psychiatry* 147:1380.

Patraglia, Felice, Fabio Facchinetti, Emelia Martignoni, Giuseppi Nappi, Annibale Volpe, and Andrea R. Genazzani (1984). "Serotonergic Agonists Increase Plasma Levels of ß-endorphin and B-lipotropin in Humans." *Journal of Clinical Endocrinology and Metabolism* 59:1138–1152.

Patterson, William (1993, February). "Fluoxetine-Induced Sexual Dysfunction." *Journal of Clinical Psychiatry* 54:71.

Paul, Steven M. (1990, April). "Serotonin and Its Effects on Human Behavior." *Journal of Clinical Psychiatry* 51 (supplement), No. 4: 3–4.

Paul, Steven M. (1993, March 9). "Why I'm Leaving Government for a Drug Firm." *Wall Street Journal* p. A18. Reprinted in *Psychiatric Times* (1993, May), p. 8.

Pennisi, E. (1994, February 26). "Seeing Synapses: New Ways to Study Nerves." *Science News* 145:135.

Physicians' Desk Reference (PDR). (1994). Montvale, N.J.: Medical Economics Data Productions Company. Published annually.

Pierson, Ransdell (1992, October). "Quayle Aids Firms That Aid the GOP." *New York Post.*

Pimsleur, J. L. (1991, May 23). "Police Say Man They Shot Used Them to Kill Himself." *San Francisco Chronicle.*

Pollack, Mark H., and Jerrold Rosenbaum (1991, January). "Fluoxetine Treatment of Cocaine Abuse in Heroin Addicts." *Journal of Clinical Psychiatry* 52:31–33.

Porrino, L. J., M. C. Ritz, N. L. Goodman, L. G. Sharpe, M. J. Kuhar, and S. R. Goldberg (1989). "Differential Effects of the Pharmacological Manipulation of Serotonin Systems on Cocaine and Amphetamine Self-Administration in Rats." *Life Sciences* 45:1529–1535.

Press-Courier (Oxnard, California), (1991, October 2). "Insanity Pleaded in Ojai Strangling," p. 1.

Psychiatric News (1994, February 4). "Another New Antidepressant Approved, Expected to Be Available by Spring," p. 2.

Psychiatric Times (1991, November). "England Bans Halcion Claiming Incomplete Drug Safety Documentation," p. 8.

Psychiatric Times (1992, September). "Study Questions Possible Link of Antidepressants to Tumor Growth," p. 1.

Public Citizen (1990, May 23). "Re: Citizens Petition for Revision of Fluoxetine (Prozac) Labeling. Letter to David Kessler, Commissioner, Food and Drug Administration." Washington, D.C.: Public Citizen.

Randrup, A., and I. Munkvad (1972). "Correlation Between Specific Effects of Amphetamines on the Brain and on Behavior." In Ellinwood, Everett H., Jr., and Sidney Cohen (eds.): *Current Concepts on Amphetamine Abuse.* Rockville, Maryland: National Institute of Mental Health. DHEW Publication No. (HMS) 72-9085. Chapter 2, pp. 17–25.

Rasmussen, Kurt, Richard A. Glennor, and George K. Aghajanian (1986). "Phenethylamine Hallucinogens in the Locus Coeruleus: Potency of Action Correlates with Rank Order of 5-HT2 Binding Affinity." *European Journal of Pharmacology* 132:79–82.

Reccoppa, Lawrence, Wendy Ann Welch, and Michael R. Ware (1990, November). "Acute Dystonia and Fluoxetine." *Journal of Clinical Psychiatry* 51:487.

Regier, Darrel A., Robert Hirshfeld, Frederick K. Goodwin, Jack D. Burke, Joyce B. Lazar, and Lewis L. Judd (1988, November). "The NIMH Depression Awareness, Recognition, and Treatment Program: Structure, Aims, and Scientific Basis." *American Journal of Psychiatry* 145:1351–1357.

Reimherr, Fred W., Mark F. Ward, and William F. Byerley (1989). "The Introductory Placebo Washout: A Retrospective Evaluation." *Psychiatric Research* 30:191–199.

Reinbrech, Steve (1991, August 24). "Dad Grieving Son's Car Death Targets Some Prescription Drugs." *Daily Local News* (Pennsylvania).

Reporter & Messenger (Rockdale, Texas) (1991, July 18). "Former Prosecutor Sues Drug Firm."

Reuters (1991, May 24). "Warning on Suicide in Prozac Use Sought." *New York Times.*

Reuters (1991, June 5). "Lilly Increases Prozac Support." *New York Times.*

Reuters (1992, November 23). "FDA's Watchdog Role Inadequate, Report Says." *Washington Post,* p. A4.

Ricaurte, G. A., R. W. Fuller, K. W. Perry, and L. S. Seiden (1983). "Fluoxetine Increases Long-Lasting Neostriatal Dopamine Depletion After Administration of D-methamphetamine and D-amphetamine." *Neuropharmacology* 22:1165–1169.

Riddle, Mark A., Robert A. King, Maureen T. Hardin, Lawrence Scahill, Sharon I. Ort, Phillip Chappell, Ann Rasmusson, and James F. Leckman (1990/1991). "Behavioral Side of Fluoxetine in Children and Adolescents." *Journal of Child and Adolescent Psychopharmacology* 1:193–198.

Rimer, Sara (1993, December 13). "With Millions Taking Prozac, a Legal Drug Culture Arises." *New York Times*, p. A1.

Rodgers, Joann Ellison (1992). *Psychosurgery: Damaging the Brain to Save the Mind.* New York: HarperCollins.

Rosen, Marty (1992, January 11). "School Reeling after 2 Suicides." *St. Petersburg Times* (Florida).

Rosenlind, Stevan (1991, July 23). "Woman Says Drug Led Her to Kill Her Mother." *Fresno Bee* (California).

Rosenlind, Stevan (1991, October 26). "Prozac Changed Defendant, Doctor Says." *Fresno Bee* (California).

Rosenthal, Elisabeth (1991, October 3). "U.S. Not Planning to Ban Sleeping Pill." *New York Times*, p. A18.

Rosenthal, Elisabeth (1994, April 10). "Maybe You're Sick. Maybe We Can Help." *New York Times*, p. 2E.

Rothman, David J. (1994, February 14). "Shiny Happy People: The Problem with 'Cosmetic Psychopharmacology.'" *New Republic*, pp. 34–38.

Rothschild, Anthony J., and Carol A. Locke (1991, December). "Reexposure to Fluoxetine After Serious Suicide Attempts By Three Patients: The Role of Akathisia." *Journal of Clinical Psychiatry* 52:491–493.

Sabshin, M. (1992, March 10). "To Aid Understanding of Mental Disorders." *New York Times*, p. A24.

Salt Lake Tribune (1991, May 14). "Utahn, 20, Dies After Fall."

Satterfield, Jamie (1991, December 5a). "Robber Fighting Depression Gets Break in Sentencing." *Mountain Press* (Sevierville, Indiana).

Scatterfield, Jamie (1991, December 5b). "Do the Advantages of Prozac Outweigh Its Disadvantages." *Mountain Press* (Sevierville, Indiana).

Scher, J. (1966). "Patterns and Profiles of Addiction and Drug Abuse." *Archives of General Psychiatry* 15:539.

Schmidt, Christopher J. (1987). "Neurotoxicity of the Psychedelic Amphetamine, Methylenedioxymethamphetamine." *Journal of Pharmacology and Experimental Therapeutics* 240:1–7.

Schwartz, John (1993, December 10). "Company Faulted in Fatal Drug Trials: Consumer Group Charges Eli Lilly Had Strong Evidence of Toxicity." *Washington Post*, p. A4.

Schwartz, Stephen (1991, November 9). "USF Professor's Pleas in Mother-Biting Case." *San Francisco Chronicle.*

Seed, J., J. Macy, P. Fleming, and A. Naess (1988). *Thinking Like a Mountain.* Philadelphia: New Society Publishers.

Settle, Edmund C., and Gina Puzzuoli Settle (1984, February). "A Case of Mania Associated with Fluoxetine." *American Journal of Psychiatry* 141:280–281.

Shear, M. Katherine, Allen Frances, and Peter Weiden (1983, August). "Suicide Associated with Akathisia and Depot Fluphenazine Treatment." *Journal of Clinical Psychopharmacology* 3:235–236.

Shenon, Philip (1985, August 22). "Lilly Pleads Guilty to Oraflex Charges." *New York Times,* P. A 16.

Sherman, Carl (1994, February). "Depression's Complex, Tangled Biologic Roots." *Clinical Psychiatry News,* p. 3.

Sherman, Carl (1994, February). "Treatment-Resistant Depression: Long List of Culprits." *Clinical Psychiatry News,* p. 14.

Slobota, Walter (1984 April 3). "Memo re John Feighner, M.D., San Diego, CA. Inspection of blanked material fluoxetine." Memo designated "NDA 18,936. (Eli Lilly)" and "For the Files." Concludes with "These observations were communicated to Paul Leber, M.D. BFN-120 on April 3, 1984." Food and Drug Administration, Department of Health and Human Services. Obtained through the Freedom of Information Act.

Smith, Roger C. (1972). "Compulsive Methamphetamine Abuse and Violence in the Haight-Ashbury District." In Ellinwood, Everett H., Jr., and Sidney Cohen (eds.): *Current Concepts on Amphetamine Abuse.* Rockville, Maryland: National Institute of Mental Health. DHEW Publication No. (HMS) 72-9085. Chapter 21, pp. 205–216.

Smith, Roger C. (1994, February 9). "Prozac: Wonder Drug for the Human Brain?" *Diamondback* (University of Maryland, College Park).

Sollmann, Torald (1943). *A Manual of Pharmacology.* Philadelphia: W. B. Saunders Company.

Song, Fujian, Nick Freemantle, Trevor A. Sheldon, Allan House, Paul Watson, Andrew Long, and James Mason (1993, March 13). "Selective Serotonin Reuptake Inhibitors: Meta-analysis of Efficacy and Acceptability." *British Medical Journal* 306:683–687.

Specter, Michael (1990, April 26). "Possible Cause of L-Tryptophan-Related Illness Found." *Washington Post,* p. A4.

Spotts, James V., and Carol A. Spotts (eds.) (1980). *Use and Abuse of Amphetamine and Its Substitutes.* Washington, D.C.: National Institute on Drug Abuse, U.S. Department of Health, Education, and Welfare. DHEW Publication No. (ADM) 80–941.

Spretnak, Charlene (1991). *States of Grace: The Recovery of Meaning in the Postmodern Age.* San Francisco: Harper-Collins.

Stark, Paul, Ray W. Fuller, and David T. Wong (1985, March). "The Pharmacological Profile of Fluoxetine." *Journal of Clinical Psychiatry* 46(3, section 2):7–13.

Stark, Paul, and C. David Hardison (1985, March). "A Review of Multicenter Controlled Studies of Fluoxetine vs. Imipramine and Placebo in Outpatients with Major Depressive Disorder." *Journal of Clinical Psychiatry* 46[3, Sec 2]:53–85.

Stein, Richard A., Murray E. Jarvik, and David A. Gorelick (1993). "Impairment of Memory by Fluoxetine in Smokers." *Experimental and Clinical Psychopharmacology* 1:188–193.

Sternbach, Harvey (1991, June). "The Serotonin Syndrome." *American Journal of Psychiatry* 148:705.

Stimmel, Glen L., Diane M. Skowron, and Walter A. Chameides (1991, August). "Focus on Fluvoxamine." *Hospital Formulary* 26:635–643.

Studwell, Gregory (1993, April 26). "Biology Professor in Jail for Beating Wife." *Meridian* (Lehman College, New York).

Styron, William (1993, January 4). "Prozac Days, Halcion Nights." *The Nation*, p. 256.

Swadish, Stacy (1991, July 31). "Testimony: Drug Caused Man's Depression." *Iowa City Press-Citizen* (Iowa).

Talbott, John A., Robert E. Hales, and Stuart C. Yudofsky (eds.) (1988). *Textbook of Psychiatry.* Washington, D.C.: American Psychiatric Press.

Tanouye, E. (1993, April 15). "Critics See Self-Interest in Lilly's Funding of Ads Telling the Depressed to Get Help." *Wall Street Journal*, p. B1.

Teicher, Martin H. (1990, November 15). Testimony in The People of the State of California, Plaintiff, vs. Mildred Johnson, Defendant. No. VA 000789. Superior Court of the State of California for the County of Los Angeles. Department Southeast F.

Teicher, Martin H., Carol A. Glod, and Jonathan O. Cole, (1990, February). "Emergence of Intense Suicidal Preoccupations

During Fluoxetine Treatment." *American Journal of Psychiatry* 147:207–210.

Teicher, Martin H., Carol A. Glod, and Jonathan O. Cole (1990, October). "Dr. Teicher and Associates Reply [to Papp and Gorman]." *American Journal of Psychiatry* 147:1380–1381.

Teicher, Martin H., Carol A. Glod, and Jonathan O. Cole (1990, November). "Dr. Teicher and Associates Reply to Miller." *American Journal of Psychiatry* 147:1572.

Teicher, Martin H., Carol A. Glod, and Jonathan O. Cole (1990, December). "Dr. Teicher and Associates Reply [to Tollefson]." *American Journal of Psychiatry* 147:1692–1693.

Teicher, Martin H., Carol A. Glod, and Jonathan O. Cole (1993). "Antidepressant Drugs and the Emergence of Suicidal Tendencies." *Drug Safety* 8(3):186–212.

Templer, Donald I., Lawrence C. Hartlage, and W. Gary Cannon (eds.) (1992). *Preventable Brain Damage.* New York: Springer Publishing Company.

Thompson, Larry (1994, March). "The Cure That Killed." *Discovery,* pp. 56–62.

Thompson, Tracy (1992, August 19). "Lead Poisoning Now Seen as Threat to More Children." *Washington Post,* p. C1.

Timmins, Annmarie (1991, December 5). "Wife Used Ax to Kill Husband." *Portsmouth Herald* (New Hampshire), p. 1.

Tobias, Andrew (1990, November 26). "Give Greed Another Chance." *Time,* p. 74.

Tollefson, Gary D. (1990, December). "Fluoxetine and Suicidal Ideation." *American Journal of Psychiatry* 147:1691–1692.

Tolliver, Thomas (1991, March 21). "Prozac Defense Used in Fayette Case." *Lexington Herald-Leader* (Kentucky).

Tork, Istvan, and Jean-Pierre Hornung (1990). "Raphe Nuclei and the Serotonergic System." In Paxinos, George (ed.): *The Human Nervous System.* New York: Academic Press. Chapter 30, pp. 1001–1022.

Touchette, Nancy (1994, February). "Biochemical Factors in Impulsive and Violent Behavior." *The Journal of NIH Research* 6:27–29.

Toups, Catherine (1991, April 29). "Bitter Pill for the Maker of Prozac." *Insight,* pp. 54–55.

Towns, Edolphus (1993, November 8). Letter from the Chairman, Subcommittee on Human Resources and Intergovernmental Relations, Committee on Government Operations, to

Margaret McCaffrey, concerning possible hearings relevant to Prozac and the FDA. Unpublished.

Turner, Dan (1991, November 5). "Final Arguments Given in Mother-Killing Trial. Medication Complicates San Jose Case." *San Francisco Chronicle.*

Turner, Samuel M., Rolf G. Jacob, Deborah C. Beidel, and Suzanne Griffin (1985, February). "A Second Case of Mania Associated with Fluoxetine." *American Journal of Psychiatry* 142:274–275.

United Press (UP) news service. (1993, January 8). "Defense Says Computer Exec 'Psychotic' When He Killed Family."

United States General Accounting Office (GAO) (1990, April). *FDA Drug Review: Postapproval Risks, 1976–1985.* Washington, D.C.: U.S. General Accounting Office.

Valentine, Paul W. (1990, March 31). "Drug Firm Admits Payoffs to FDA Regulators." *Washington Post,* p. A15.

Vosburgh, Glenda (1991, September 19). "Baby Survives Shooting." *Parks Cities People* (Dallas, Texas).

Waldholz, Michael (1990, July 18). "Prozac Said to Spur Idea of Suicide." *Wall Street Journal,* p. B4.

Walker, Parks W., Jonathan O. Cole, Elmer A. Gardner, Arlene R. Hughes, Andrew Johnson, Sharyn R. Batey, and Charles G. Lineberry (1993, December). "Improvement in Fluoxetine-Associated Sexual Dysfunction in Patients Switched to Buproprion." *Journal of Clinical Psychiatry* 54:459–465.

Wamsley, James K., William F. Byerley, R. Tyler McCabe, Elizabeth J. McConnell, Ted M. Dawson, and Bernard I. Grosser (1987). "Receptor Alterations Associated with Serotonergic Agents: An Autographic Analysis." *Journal of Clinical Psychiatry* 48(3, Supplement):19–85.

Weiner, William J., and Elliot D. Luby (1983, November). "Tardive Akathisia." *Journal of Clinical Psychiatry* 44:417–419.

Welner, S. A., C. de Montigny, J. Desroches, P. Desjardins, and B. E. Suranyi-Cadotte (1989). *Synapse* 4:347–352.

Wilcox, James Allen (1987, August). "Abuse of Fluoxetine by a Patient with Anorexia Nervosa." *American Journal of Psychiatry* 144:1100.

Wirshing, William C., Theodore van Putten, James Rosenberg, Stephen Marder, Donna Ames, and Tara Hicks-Gray (1992, July). "Fluoxetine, Akathisia, and Suicidality: Is There a Causal Connection." *Archives of General Psychiatry* 49:580–581.

Wise, Dean (1991, August 23). "Grieving Father Eyes Reform, Not Revenge." *York Daily Record* (Pennsylvania), p. 1.

Wohl, Stanley (1984). *The Medical Industrial Complex*. New York: Harmony Books.

Wong, David T., and Frank P. Bymaster (1981, April). "Subsensitivity of Serotonin Receptors After Long-Term Treatment of Rats with Fluoxetine." *Research Communications in Chemical Pathology and Pharmacology* 32:41–51.

Wong, David T., Jong S. Horng, Frank P. Bymaster, Kenneth L. Hauser, and Bryan B. Molloy (1974). "A Selective Inhibitor of Serotonin Uptake: Lilly 110140, 3-(p-trifluoromethylphenoxy)-N-methyl-3-phenylpropylamine." *Life Sciences* 15: 471–479.

Wong, D. T., L. R. Reid, F. P. Bymaster, and Penny G. Threlkeld (1985). "Chronic Effects of Fluoxetine, a Selective Inhibitor of Sertonin Up-take, on Neurotransmitter Receptors." *Journal of Neural Transmission* 64:251–269.

World Health Organization Expert Committee on Addiction-Producing Drugs (1957). *WHO Technical Report Series,* 116.

Yu, Dianna S. L., Forrest L. Smith, Doris G. Smith, and William H. Lyness (1986). "Fluoxetine-Induced Attenuation of Amphetamine Self-Administration in Rats." *Life Sciences* 39: 1383–1388.

Index

About the Authors

Peter R. Breggin, M.D., is an internationally known psychiatrist in private practice in Bethesda, Maryland. He is the founder and director of the nonprofit Center for the Study of Psychiatry, which includes *Children First!*, the only membership organization devoted to protecting children and families from biopsychiatric intrusions into their lives. He is also professor of conflict resolution at George Mason University and the author of many books and articles, most recently *Toxic Psychiatry* (1991) and *Beyond Conflict* (1992), both published by St. Martin's Press.

Dr. Breggin's reform work began in the 1950s as a Harvard College student when he directed the Harvard-Radcliffe Mental Hospital Volunteer Program. He received his medical training at Case Western Reserve and his psychiatric training at Harvard and the State University of New York, Upstate Medical Center. Before going into private practice in 1968, he was a full-time consultant with the National Institute of Mental Health. During the 1970s, he won recognition for organizing a successful campaign against the return of lobotomy and then went on to write the first medical books about the brain-damaging effects of electroshock and psychiatric drug treatment.

Dr. Breggin continues to influence the mental health professions through his private practice, workshops, publications, research, and medical-legal activities. His reform efforts have been extensively covered in the general and scientific press from the *New York Times* and *Time* magazine to *Science* magazine and the *New Scientist.* Among many media appearances, he has been a psychiatric expert on *60 Minutes, 20/20,* and *Dan Rather Reports.*

Ginger Ross Breggin is Director for Research and Education at the Center for the Study of Psychiatry. In 1992 she initiated and spearheaded the national campaign against the federal violence initiative, including funding for a conference on "Genetic Factors in Crime," and has recently helped to set up *Children First!* Her background is in public relations, writing, and investigative journalism. She works closely with Dr. Breggin in all of the center's activities and has coauthored articles in the fields of mental health and conflict resolution. She is also an award-winning photographer and a mother. This is her first published book.